Becoming an Exceptional AAC Leader

Inspiration from 15 Augmentative and Alternative Communication Champions

With Foreword by Alan Brightman

www.MaiLingChan.com

Mai Ling Chan, LLC
Phoenix, AZ

Table of Contents

Foreword

By Alan Brightman, PhD

"The universe is made of stories, not of atoms." [1]

- Muriel Rukeyser

"To love what you do and feel that it matters, how could anything be more fun?" [2]

- Katherine Graham

* * *

It was dark when I landed at San Francisco International Airport in July of 1984. I rented a car to drive the hour or so it would take me to get to my destination. The interior light bulb was dim, making my wrestling with the wrinkled paper map increasingly frustrating. The map, incidentally, didn't talk. It didn't announce which way to turn in 700 feet. It never told me it was "recalculating." But it got me to the motel. Just a convenient mile from the place where I was to work for the next 13 years.

I had accepted a new job at what was then called Apple Computer (today simply known as Apple), which meant that I

[1] "Muriel Rukeyser Quotes." BrainyQuote.com. BrainyMedia Inc, 2021. 22 March 2021. https://www.brainyquote.com/quotes/muriel_rukeyser_131826

[2] "Katharine Graham Quotes." BrainyQuote.com. BrainyMedia Inc, 2021. 22 March 2021. https://www.brainyquote.com/quotes/katharine_graham_126094

was leaving behind years of work in the nonprofit sector working mostly in the areas of disability awareness, advocacy, and education. Aside from summer jobs mowing lawns, lining little league fields, and crafting obscenely unhealthy ice cream sundaes and banana splits, this would be my first real full-time job. Now I'd be part of a big, growing corporation, a company whose founder was seemingly in the national headlines every day and on the covers of magazines ranging from *Fortune* to *Mad Magazine*. Steve Jobs. Brilliant. Arrogant. Uniquely newsworthy. Endlessly quotable.

Yes, this was the company that was, for the first time in history, creating computer products for "the rest of us," adults and kids alike. So, it didn't take much persuading to get me to move from coast to coast. I couldn't wait to experience the Apple excitement firsthand.

The next morning, I walked onto the campus of Apple Computer. Sunny, alive, and green. Several small, animated groups huddled on the grass. Impromptu meetings maybe? Three jugglers. Torn jeans, shorts, and t-shirts. A guy riding a unicycle. A girl riding a unicycle. Rock music coming from a place I couldn't see. More rock music coming from the parking garage. One would be excused for thinking he'd just walked into the first day of clown school, but this was Apple Computer in 1984—an environment like nothing I'd experienced ever before.

With all there was to see and hear, one thing caught my eye indelibly. Almost everywhere I looked, I saw people wearing caps and clothes emblazoned with six words: *A computer can change your life*. Posters and bumper stickers displayed the same message: *A computer can change your life.*

I didn't get it.

For years I had been in the business of trying to make some lives a little better, maybe even changing a few. But I was doing so from the nonprofit world where, for example, if people were hungry, nobody made catchy slogans. Everybody instead made sandwiches.

A computer can change your life. It was everywhere. Just a slogan. But on this campus, true believers were all around me.

I really didn't get it.

In fact, the slogan caused me to think about something else entirely. If, in fact, a computer can change your life, I wondered, doesn't that actually say more about your life than about a computer? What kind of a life must one have, I questioned, if it could be changed simply by a plastic box, a keyboard, and a screen?

I was certainly not a believer on that first day.

I would become a believer though, a proselytizer, in less than a year.

Because I began to see for myself how the personal computer was, in fact, changing lives, especially the lives of kids and adults with disabilities. I even began to see how the computer might be able to actually—fundamentally— change *the experience of being disabled*. Seeing this led me to create Apple's Worldwide Disability Solutions Group.

Over the years, I know the work we did at Apple changed some lives. The lives, themselves, made that dramatically clear.

Today, of course, personal electronics and their wide-ranging impact are commonplace to the point where a teenage girl, who several years ago was participating in a study designed to suggest new cell phone features, announced that "Nothing amazes me anymore." (Yeah, I know. Pathetic in lots of ways. But I knew what she meant.) (I should immediately and unabashedly add that I continue to be amazed by technology every day.)

Let me give you just one example of what I mean by personal computers changing the experience of disability.

By all accounts, Johnny was a uniquely talented jazz musician, but at age 21, he was involved in a tragic car accident that left him unable to move anything below his neck. In live performances and on his recordings, he had relied on his fingers to create and communicate his music. He could no longer use a keyboard.

At the rehab center where Johnny spent considerable time following the accident, he was asked, "What do you want to be now? What would you like to be able to do?" The questions were irrelevant to him. "It's not what I want to be now," he'd answer. "It's who I am. It's who I've always been. I'm a jazz musician."

Because they saw he was an artist, and because they were certain he'd never be able to play music again, the rehab folks tried things like putting colored pencils or paintbrushes in his mouth. "Here's a new artistic way to express yourself," they offered. "Try this." Johnny would have none of it.

"I don't draw. I don't paint. I'm a jazz musician."

Sometime after he left the rehab center, my team and I were introduced to Johnny and were eager to see whether any of Apple's personal computer technologies might help him get a little closer to becoming again, who he always was.

Two years later, at the annual convention of the American Occupational Therapy Association, Johnny rolled onstage to the polite but uncertain applause of the thousand members who'd come to hear our Keynote address. He positioned himself in front of a Macintosh computer. He had a stick in his mouth, and he pressed a key.

Music started. *His* music. Music that he had written and that he was now playing live.

What had been uncertain applause among the attendees was quickly replaced with lively toe tapping and finger snapping. And raucous, noisy sounds of "More!"

Johnny was Johnny again.

Until he passed away at much too young an age, Johnny made a point of regularly sending audio recordings of his music—*his* music—back to his old rehab center. It mattered to him that the people there understood what he had known all along: no one is entitled to impose a ceiling on someone else's potential.

Because of the personal computer, Johnny was able to continue to be who he knew he was. Even if others had their doubts. In glorious sounds and with not a single word, Johnny screamed to the excited attendees, "I'm a jazz musician."

More than 150 years ago, the popular British essayist, Walter Bagehot, wrote something that describes Johnny's journey tellingly. "The great pleasure in life," he wrote, "is doing what people say you cannot do."

As you'll see in the pages of this book, Johnny is not the only person who's used assistive technology—and perseverance—to complete a life-changing personal journey.

* * *

This book doesn't set out to teach you a thing; instead, it introduces you to people telling often intimate stories about themselves and others and about practices and experiences that matter to them. Just as with Johnny's story, there is no explicit intent to tell you what you should learn. No steps to take to make you a better anything. Each in their own way, the authors invite you to become familiar with an aspect of their lives that centers around communication, in general, and augmentative and alternative communication (AAC) in particular.

What you take away from these encounters will be impressions from the people you meet, not learnings from a curriculum. You'll meet mentors and those they've mentored. You'll meet people who don't talk about doing. They simply just do. And you'll meet people who exude a passion for their work that exemplifies what Emily Dickinson described as "a phosphorescence for learning."[3]

Present throughout these pages are people with and without disabilities. Not remarkable people. Not heroic people. Just

[3] Kirkby, Joan. *Emily Dickinson*. Macmillan International Higher Education 1993, pp. 4

people. Real ones.

* * *

It's been said that great photographers have learned to *listen to the light*.

Imagine that. Imagine hearing something when there is no sound. I think of this sometimes when I'm with someone who isn't able to speak. Even before she interacts with whatever communication tool she's using, I find myself *listening* to her. Listening to all the indications of communication even when no formal communication has yet taken place. Sound contradictory? Maybe even a little goofy? Well maybe. But as you'll see when you meet the people in this book, communication, itself, means more than the words one speaks.

Listen to the light.

My Community

Listen to my interview on the Xceptional Leaders Podcast with Mai Ling Chan

Ways to Connect with Me

LinkedIn: www.linkedin.com/in/abrightman/

Alan Brightman received a PhD in education from Harvard University and an honorary PhD in science from The University of Massachusetts. His professional accomplishments in areas related to individuals with disabilities as well as older adults reflect a career devoted both to increasing the quality of life for underserved and too-often overlooked members of society and to developing large-scale business opportunities to serve the needs of these segments. Brightman was the founder of Apple Computer's Worldwide Disability Solutions Group and served as its director for 13 years and most recently a vice president at Yahoo, where he created the Accessibility Group in 2006. Brightman's book, *DisabilityLand*, was the recipient of a Benjamin Franklin Award.

Acknowledgements

First and foremost, I thank my husband Cameron, and my children, Nick, Alex, and Raegan, for their endless support and encouragement. We have one more book to launch in this series and I'm going to continue to need your love and positivity!

I also thank my mom, Rosalba Chan, for helping me believe I can accomplish anything I put my positive, heart-felt energy toward.

A deep, heartfelt thank you goes to each and every author for taking time out of their busy lives to reflect on the events and experiences that shaped them into the person they are today. Identifying and acknowledging the importance of these moments was a crucial first step, and I am grateful to you for sharing intimate conversations and emotions that deepened and enriched the shared experiences with you.

Everyone asks me how I accomplish so much. The answer is, "respect and support from my business partners." I specifically thank Andreas Forsland (CEO and cofounder, Cognixion), Pradeesh Thomas (CEO and cofounder, Verge Learning), and all my team members at each company, for understanding the deep value of the projects and offerings I choose to dedicate my time to.

This book was definitely one that *took a village*. I am very grateful to many AAC experts, professionals, colleagues, and people who use AAC who were open to conversations with me as I created and materialized the mission and vision of this offering. I humbly look forward to the feedback and opportunities for the book to be shared far beyond my initial ideas.

Becoming an Exceptional AAC Leader

Many people have touched my life and made me want to be more knowledgeable, more helpful, more effective, more prepared—*more* of anything needed to help them have a happier and more fulfilling life. I include Xochitl's photo, with the approval of her mom, in my chapter because she is a perfect example of someone who always reminded me that happiness comes from within. Her constant smile and gentle touch effectively communicate her beautiful and loving spirit. AAC is simply a tool to put words to what is in her heart.

Always a phone call, text, or email away, I thank the people who haven't deleted me from their contacts yet: Matt Chan, Lori DiBlasi, Laura Stevenson, Patrick G. Poli, Thomas McDowell, Mary Huston, and my podcast hubby, Martyn Sibley.

The final version of the book took five months to assemble and I am forever grateful to my amazing, international team of experts: Jennifer Baljko—developmental editor; Cori Wamsley and Allison Hrip—final editors; Christie Mayer—book cover; Jeren Calinisan—social media; and Angela Smith—content design. You help bring our stories together as a collective and unified offering.

Introduction

This second book in the *Becoming an Exceptional Leader* series focuses on sharing first-person stories as they relate to assistive technology for communication. The first of its kind for this community, the collective chapters represent humanity's commitment to the ultimate achievement of universal access to communication and the elimination of related marginalization. These intimate life journeys invite you to deepen your personal connection with augmentative and alternative communication (AAC) and join the global call to action.

Coauthor voices include People who use AAC, parents, assistive technology experts, and speech-language pathologists—people who are all passionately connected by their reverence for the beauty of human interaction. And, yes, I mean "People" with a capital "P" who use AAC as a way to bring more awareness to the simple fact that they are people first and foremost, and above all else.

This group of coauthors is also united in their dedication to the continued growth and progress of the discipline as a whole, in addition to related research, funding, education, and all efforts focused on individualism and connection.

To understand the full value of this book, it is essential to define how three key words represent the mission: AAC, leader, and champion.

What is AAC? Simply put, this encompasses all the possibilities available for a person to be able to send a unique communication message. This ranges from a smile, gesture, or touching a tablet computer to the advanced interaction with electromagnetic brain waves. Strategies and delivery methods are tools used to enhance the effectiveness of the exchange, but people are ultimately the producers and the receivers of the words and messages. They are the shepherds of this intimate human interaction.

Although it has been within the realm of speech-language pathology for approximately 70 years[4], AAC has origins back to visual messages used by Ancient Greece in the 19th Century when sign language was first introduced. Since then, alternative communication has extended to auditory (Morse code) and visual (communication symbols and text) systems. The delivery of these options has also evolved as technology has become more innovative and accessible. The one constant throughout this transformation has been the need for individuals to assume direct involvement in the progression and expansion of these options. All stakeholders, including People who use AAC, parents, communication partners, support personnel, researchers, and clinicians, have all played a consistent role in the continuous evolution of this area of human communication.

It is important to share the incredible growth made within this niche area of communication to understand the significance of each contributing author of this book. When I began discussing this anthology with people in the AAC community, they immediately understood the vision and value it offered.

[4] Beukelman, D. R., & Light, J. C. (2020). *Augmentative and Alternative Communication: Supporting children and adults with complex communication needs* (5th ed.). Baltimore: MD: Brookes Publishing Co.

But there was also a request to ensure all voices would be represented and not limited to a purely professional or educational viewpoint. This was always my intention, and I am honored to include personal stories from a wide range of people invested in the future of AAC. This is where the term *leader* comes in.

As with every community, there are so many people who have demonstrated dedication and passion to the advancement of all areas of AAC, that it was quite difficult to assume the responsibility of selecting only a few representatives. With the help of notable and personally invested AAC representatives, I identified a collection of high-impact achievers that, when woven together, reflect the recent history of AAC's progress. They each contribute to the collective growth, and their individual vision and actions are significant.

"A leader is best when people barely know he exists, when his work is done, his aim fulfilled, they will say: we did it ourselves."[5] - Lao Tzu

Each coauthor I invited immediately agreed to participate, but they all had the same question, "Why me? What will I write about?" I share this with you to set the tone for the stories you are about to read. Every author is so very humble and regards their contribution as their service, not their accomplishment. They graciously accepted my invitation to share their personal story of *Becoming an Exceptional AAC Leader*.

---

[5] Oxford Essential Quotations. Ed. Ratcliffe, Susan. Oxford University Press, 2018. Oxford Reference. Date Accessed 23 Mar. 2021 <https://www.oxfordreference.com/view/10.1093/acref/9780191866692.001.0001/acref-9780191866692>.

Although their schedules were already full, they found ways to carve out dedicated writing time, and they embraced the intimate writing process with the goal of connecting with and inspiring *you*. I met with each one individually as well as in a group to review the outline and initial writing prompts, and then the writing process began.

A few may disagree with me, but I believe this was a very different writing experience than most of the coauthors had ever experienced. Because I asked them to approach it in a memoir style, there is a deeper level of vulnerability that is essential to the final product. This is a presentation style we don't often use in our professional or public communication. I admit I also struggled with this in my personal chapter in the first book of this series and started to dread the writing process for my chapter in this book. But in the end, I embraced the initial hesitancy and doubt, and wrote what I believed would be beneficial to you and other readers. I can proudly say that every coauthor has also accomplished this in their individual chapter, and every story offers a genuine connection with the person behind the words.

It is important to remember that this is an anthology, and each person has a very different style of communicating. We set out with the deliberate intention to honor the authenticity of their experience and their voice, and we hope we achieved that aim.

As you will read in the following chapters, each coauthor has experienced a unique journey to personal growth as it relates to this very specific area of communication. Their personal spirit, courage, resilience, and creativity are the secret sauce of their progressive journeys, but their steadfast commitment to *every person's right to connect and be heard* is the heart of their work. Ultimately, they are each affected by AAC in one way or another and connected to each other by their commitment to this purpose.

This is where the word *champion* in the sub-title of this book is relevant. Rather than the sports definition, which encapsulates the idea of winning at something, we use champion to mean advocating and fighting on behalf of another person. This is the core of every coauthor's being, service, and life's work. Such values are evident in first-person accounts of experiencing life with communication differences; capturing attention and spotlighting needs as a result of personal accomplishments or advocacy; designing products based on personal experience; educating from an intimate lived-experience; and, above all, demanding equality, respect, and the elimination of stereotypes and misconceptions.

The creation of novel tools and resources has also been essential to several of the coauthors, as shared by a father's decision to redirect his career skills to advocacy and product development; stories about the many years of professional dedication to abundant and highly respected online resources; and the creation and support for AAC dedicated communities, digital information, individual spotlights, and development of high-tech technology.

In addition, essential foundational supports are represented in the stories by language development experts, researchers, and online educators—all dedicated to the support, growth, and continued success of the individual who uses AAC to communicate.

Most importantly, in absolute respect for "Nothing for us without us," we are honored to share the very personal stories from our coauthors who use some type of alternative means of communication. They are all unique in their methods of access and choice of technology, yet generous with their personal stories and what they wanted to share with you.

It is our collective wish that our stories provide perspective, insight, and inspiration, and we invite you to join us in service to the AAC community.

The world continues to need new, more, and different ways to foster genuine and sincere interpersonal communications. It's up to each of us to choose how we speak, how we want to be heard, and how to fully express our individual gifts and talents.

What choice will you make?

Challenges Demand Creativity: Teaming Up to Close AAC Gaps

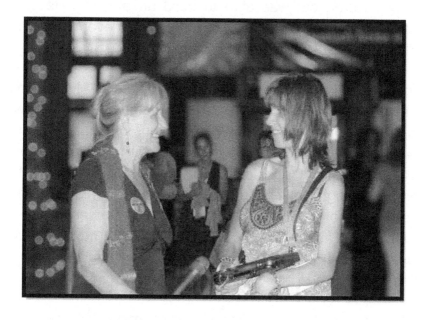

Dr. Caroline Ramsey Musselwhite, MS, CCC-SLP

* * *

My home was a bit different from those of my friends.

First, it was the chief hangout *space* in the neighborhood; then, later, in the town. There were always people around. If the cheerleaders needed a place for a slumber party, my home was instantly volunteered. When aspiring poets needed a venue, my home—the only one named after a poem ("Innisfree")—became the place for poetry recitations over dinner.

But, the most influential factor of my home was my dad. He had been totally blinded during World War II. He never saw his wife or children but was able to build an amazing life as a small-town lawyer—and also build the best-ever doghouse and the coolest ping pong table around.

It was the late 1950s, and times were different. My dad told me he had to be a much better lawyer than the others in town because people had such low expectations of him. Observing his interactions with strangers reinforced this early awareness of the treatment of people with disabilities. I remember, for example, being at a restaurant for dinner one night (a very special occasion for my family) and watching the server turn to my Mom and ask, "What does HE want?" My mother never skipped a beat, and she responded, "I don't have a clue. I guess you'll have to ask him."

This generalization of disability—assuming because he couldn't see he couldn't hear, speak or make choices—was so obvious, and so frustrating that it made a huge impact on me. I became more aware of the concept of disability, which was rarely talked about at the time. But more importantly, growing up with my dad helped me to see that his disability was a small part of his personality, though it had an impact on his life and work.

Though I didn't recognize it at the time, this early awareness of the difference of abilities encouraged me in high school to become a volunteer tutor for students with significant literacy struggles. Then in college, I volunteered at a state institution for people with intellectual disabilities. When I signed up again my sophomore year, they made me the head of volunteers because up until then, I was told, "no one has ever come back," and I was asked to work on the non-ambulatory ward.

It was a grim place, with about 16 large metal beds with high sides. Each week I visited Cheryl, a young woman about my age who was blind and had significant motor impairments because of hydrocephaly. She was a great conversationalist and loved to go to the sunroom to feel the sun on her face and have some private time. One November, she asked me to include her friend Linda, who lived in the same ward but didn't have an actual wheelchair. A kind custodian had rigged a moveable chair by attaching a canvas chair to a piece of plywood on four casters. It was tricky, and slow, pulling Cheryl and pushing Linda, but we made it work.

To my 19-year-old eyes, Linda had no clear means of communication, and I assumed she probably didn't understand our conversations. I was about to find out just how wrong I was!

One day, I arrived to find Linda crying and thought she was ill. Cheryl explained, "Oh no, she's upset because Derek on Days of Our Lives died today. We thought he was going to make it."

It turned out that Cheryl and Linda had developed a system. Linda could see the clock but couldn't verbalize her request;

each afternoon at 2 p.m., she began yelling with increasing volume. Cheryl reminded the staff to change the channel to Linda's favorite soap opera if they wanted any peace. Teamwork!

This changed my view of Linda and reminded me that I had done exactly what people had done to my Dad—made unfounded conclusions about his abilities with minimal information. I truly wish I could report that I made an effective communication system for Linda, but it was 1971 and I didn't yet have the knowledge or the skills to create that support system. But, I treated Linda with the respect and interaction that she—and everyone—deserves. My experience with her and at that state institution led me to change my major to speech-language pathology so I could begin the journey of figuring out how to better help people like Linda.

It's a tough journey, and I still have a long way to go, but challenges demand creativity.

My Biggest Challenges

I learned many life lessons while being a doctoral student.

My husband and I lived in West Virginia, about a 90-minute drive from the university, then add at least 30 minutes to find parking! It snowed almost every day in winter. Students used the unpaved lot, so my car got stuck at least once a week. And I was pregnant, so I definitely was not able to push my car. My mentor Ken helped me more than once. As a powerfully independent feminist, I learned the lesson that we all need help sometimes—and that's okay.

I also learned a great lesson in humility. I had done really well in my coursework and aced my written exams. At the same time, I was also writing my first textbook, so I didn't study enough for my orals (which covered 13 areas of study, with a seven-member team asking rapid-fire questions.) By the end of the two hours, I don't think I could have told them my name. So, when the department chair asked if I'd like to continue the orals after the holiday, with much relief, I left the meeting and went home to study— for eight weeks.

It was a tough eight weeks of 12-hour study days fueled by junk food and support from my husband, friends, and children. But I learned how to deeply research tough topics, organize my notes for a quick review, and prepare oral arguments with minimal fear. As a result, I aced the orals and moved forward with my dissertation.

When we moved to the mountains of North Carolina in the early 80s, I got a great job as the speech-language pathologist for a private, nonprofit center for students with significant disabilities. It was a wonderful place to work, but there were several significant challenges.

Funding was a *huge* challenge. I was the head of the speech-language department (meaning that I was the only SLP) with an annual budget of $50 for materials. We were constantly in fundraising mode. While this felt daunting at the time, it helped me learn to write small grants. I got so good at writing and promoting them that we went from zero student computers to multiple computers in each room, plus a plethora of software. We also started a lending library of adapted devices and toys, and we even built an amazing adapted playground. We did all this with grants ranging from $500 to $5000. I became so skilled at writing grants, that I even wrote a book on *Mini Grants and Volunteers!*

Finding adapted materials was another obstacle as we didn't have color printers for communication displays, switch mounts, or even enough switches for our students. We got creative and figured out how to barter for materials and time.

For instance, I bartered:

- My time doing monthly disability awareness talks to a 6th-grade class in exchange for an annual toy drive; coloring in black and white 'big books' that were more engaging for my students and visiting bi-annually. (I found out later that a number of these 6th graders had gone to college to study special education, and train to become speech/language, occupational, or physical therapists.)
- My time working with Scout troops in exchange for learning electronics to make switches (to operate battery toys or electrical appliances such as blenders) and switch adapters (small gadgets to connect the handmade switches to the toys); color backgrounds for communication displays and make dolls with disabilities for an awareness project.
- My time as a speaker for adult service clubs in exchange for volunteers to copy software floppy disks containing material we had created, create choice boards, and be 1:1 readers.

We got creative in other ways, too. My own children volunteered their time to color pages, help set up communication devices that would speak for our students, use special software programs to create new activities for my students, and use special tools to bind books that I sold. In exchange, I became their Scout Leader and took them and their friends on special day trips.

These opportunities became chapters on volunteering and bartering in my 1985 book, *Adaptive Play,* and the project plans for many of the items we built were included in the *Project Planbook* series completed in the 1990s.

Insufficient staff was also an ongoing issue. I was the only SLP for about 50 students with significant disabilities, most of whom needed AAC—and I was only half time! Eventually, we had the help of a graduate student each year, but they needed significant supervision. We just needed another certified SLP. So, I made a deal with the director: If I could raise half the money for the salary, he would match it. The gauntlet was thrown!

We started a Parent-to-Parent group at the center, and the parents agreed to host a three-day conference if I would be the speaker. Parents cooked all of the food (we ended up selling a cookbook!) and they created materials to sell, found a free space for the event, and handled registrations. On a budget of $500, we raised $15,000 each year for three years! It was exhausting but we were raising awareness, as well as funds. Out of that grew the annual AAC in the Desert conference in Phoenix.

Each of these challenges forced us to think outside the box to find workable solutions. They also led to powerful life lessons for me and sometimes to strategies that could be shared with others through workshops, books, and software.

My Gifts

Connecting with people has been my greatest gift, and it has taken many forms over the past 45 years.

Mentoring has been incredibly important to me. I had several wonderful mentors early in my journey and vowed to pay it forward. I have been lucky to work with scores of graduate students, beginning teachers, and others who share my passions about AAC and literacy. I have also been fortunate to have long-term connections with people who use AAC and their families. I am currently working with people I have known for at least 25 years. We know that our best learning as professionals is from those connections, but I have found that seeing progress and struggles over time has been incredibly insightful as well, and helped me share the deep lessons I continue to learn.

For the past 25 years, I have also actively sought ways to help people who use AAC develop social interactions.

As an example, Speech-Language Pathologist Jan Pilling, and I, started a social communication program called Communication Circles in the 1990s to support individuals who needed both support and connections with their typical peers. Peers learn to model with the student's AAC system, and it also helps to facilitate both communication and friendships. This has mushroomed to include thousands of Communication Circles across the world.

In another project, dating back to the late 1990s, Deanna Wagner, a speech-language pathologist, and I started Out and About, a community outing group for people who use AAC and their families and friends. Krista Howard, one of the coauthors of this book (read Krista's story on page 130), was initially a member of the group, but when she was about 15 years old, she used her device to tell me that we needed a group closer to home, and she wanted to help run it. Since then, Out and About has expanded beyond Arizona with scores of groups around the world.

Another one of my greatest gifts is finding partners. My family are my original partners, from my husband who provided incredible support throughout grad school and continues today, to my children who volunteered (and were sometimes "voluntold"), to my sister and cousins who often met me on the road. Many of my books and presentations are collaborative efforts with partners such as Gretchen, undertaken in creative ways, like brainstorming sessions in cars and trains, during snowstorms, and on thinking walks with some of my coauthors and co-creators.

My Wish for You

I hope you can connect creatively with others on a similar journey—and *stay* connected. Seeing the waves of growth in the lives of AAC and literacy learners can help all of us provide significantly better support to people who use AAC and to their families.

Always remember that when we are interacting with any learners, the goal is: "Down with demands, up with invitations!"

Recommendations

- **Think ahead.** Don Johnston—the founder and CEO of the company that bears his name—has shown a deep commitment to ensuring that literacy for all truly means <u>all</u>. I've known him for 40 years and he asked me decades ago where I saw myself in 5, 10, or 15 years. I didn't start truly planning ahead until my 60s. But now that I am more proactive, my journey has become even more exciting.
- **Figure out your life-work balance early.** We want you here for the long haul and not to burn out early!
- **Choose your focus.** My themes include literacy (including the power of poetry), supporting friendships through Communication Circles and Out & About, and figuring out ways to have FUN while learning.
- **Find your partners.** Remember that you can enjoy partner power anywhere, including getting pedicures, hiking, kayaking, and floating in a pool!

My Community

Watch my interview with Mai Ling Chan on Cognixion's What's New? What's Next? in AAC:

Website: www.aacintervention.com

Blog: https://aacgirls.blogspot.com/

TeachersPayTeachers:
www.teacherspayteachers.com/Store/Caroline-Musselwhite

(Be sure to download the free Out and About book)

Ways to Connect with Me

Pinterest: (see especially AAC & Literacy Quotes) www.pinterest.com/carolinemussel/aac-lit-quotes/

Twitter: @AACCaroline

Instagram: @carolineramseymusselwhite and @poetrypoweraac

Dr. Caroline Musselwhite is an assistive technology specialist with more than 45 years of experience working with children and adolescents with significant disabilities in a variety of settings. Dr. Musselwhite has written a number of textbooks and instructional books on a range of topics and has authored many books and software programs for youth with disabilities. She has taught courses at several universities and presented thousands of workshops throughout North and South America, Australia, Europe, and Africa. Honors include Educator of the Year (Association for Retarded Citizens, NC), DiCarlo Outstanding Clinician Award (NC Speech-Language-Hearing Association), and ISAAC Fellow.

An Unexpected Life

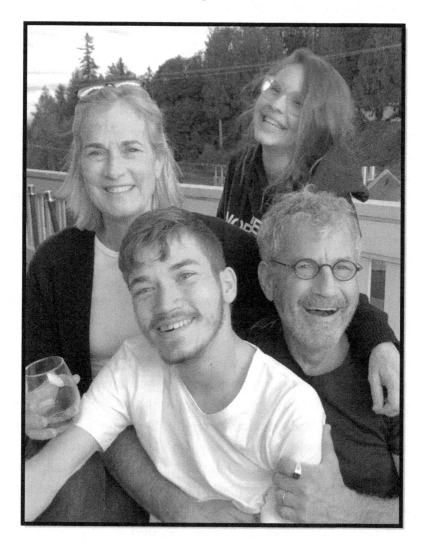

Richard Ellenson, Parent

* * *

I was an advertising creative executive, born out of a college English major, sprinkled with decent fiction and slightly better wine. I began my career at the large New York agencies, then started my own creative boutique. I wrote "It's Not TV. It's HBO," often thought of as one of media's most enduring taglines. I produced big, fun commercials for world-renowned brands such as American Express, Kellogg's, and McDonald's. I got to build sets like a full-sized facade of the White House. I visited the chateau where they create Cointreau liquor, attended the Paris Air Show with the CEO of Saab Aircraft, and traveled the backroads of Mexico's Yucatan to meet dozens of indigenous children and learn about their lives for a print campaign. And all the while, I was lucky enough to be immersed in the buzz and thrum of New York City, with its hard-charging ambition and cultural brilliance.

Then, in September 1997, my son, Tom, was born with cerebral palsy.

Tom, my wonderful son, would turn out to be a bright, determined, and charming person, who would require a power wheelchair for mobility and an augmentative and alternative communication (AAC) device to speak. During his early years, I learned the world of disability had so many remarkable individuals committed to helping us: speech language pathologies, assistive technology professionals, teachers, caregivers, and, heaven knows, incredible parents. However, what it didn't have was someone steeped in marketing and design, who's first thought was not to address the issues of the condition, but instead, to address the perceptions surrounding it.

Over the next 23 years, I turned my passion for storytelling and communication toward my son's world, determined to use all I had experienced to change what I felt was one of the most complex, difficult, and least understood brands in the world: disability.

In advertising, one looks to capture what the world will find compelling. Certainly, the early years of a child's severe cerebral palsy are challenging. But they are also filled with the beautiful moments: moments of learning, of exploration, days outside in a park, inside giggling at TV videos, days watching a child's curiosity delight at others: watching one's son's desire to achieve, his sense of appreciation, his smile. I realized almost immediately that I would not be one who'd fall into sadness about my son's disability; rather, I was drawn to discover all there would be to embrace, enjoy, and share as his life unfolded. As Tom's father, I was determined to set an example that would support his belief in himself, and help him grow into the person he would one day imagine himself to be.

In my advertising career, I had become well-versed in communication strategies that shift perceptions in 30 seconds. In my field's close proximity to Hollywood, I had seen wildly cool technology, from computer-generated imagery to audio transformations. In working with graphic artists, I'd been taught the enormous impact and influence of design. And as I looked out over the terrain of what would be my son's future, I was determined to bring all this insight to his world: a world which so desperately needed new language, new images, and changed perceptions.

Becoming an Exceptional AAC Leader

Here are a few things that happened along the way.

* * *

In 2003, as we were trying to find an appropriate kindergarten for Tom, we ran into New York City Mayor Mike Bloomberg at a restaurant. As the mayor walked by our table, I got up, introduced myself, and shared my concerns. It was an impromptu ad pitch, if you will. I told him I had heard there was not an appropriate inclusive program in the city's schools. I told him we needed to start something new.

The mayor gave me his card and told me to call the next day.

If this were a longer chapter, I'd tell the entire story, but here's the short version. The mayor gave his personal support and opened doors: doors I had to go through myself where I would visit dozens of pre-Ks and find amazing children to fill the inclusive program we were creating. Tom's years in the NYC public schools were hard and certainly not perfect. We were always educating the educators. Tom was always blazing trails. It was exhausting and frustrating. But it was good.

Tom's first year in the NYC school system became a cover story in the *New York Times Sunday Magazine*. Wow! But even more importantly, that story ended fourteen years later, with Tom enrolling at SUNY/Purchase as a freshman, majoring in theater and arts management. He was the first student ever to use a power wheelchair and augmentative communication, as he brought his determined spirit, love for performance, and desire to achieve to that campus.

Fate is funny. Sometimes it tells you what to do. Sometimes it hollers. Tom's education happened because I was eating at the same restaurant as the mayor of New York right as we were having trouble finding a school for my son. I stood up out of an instinct borne of desperation, and I became an accidental advocate. But what I learned in that moment is that people want to help. It's just that, so often, they don't know how. When you can do, show others what they can do. You can't demand karma. But when you stumble upon it, pick it up, and do what it tells you to do. Be an accidental advocate.

* * *

Cerebral palsy (CP) is a condition with enormous variation. It can simply affect one's gait or balance, impair one's grasp or speech in a minor way, or it can create deeply significant physical and intellectual challenges, including severe challenges to hearing, sight, speaking, and intellectual ability.

Tom's CP, though not rare, is less typical. He has a bright, engaging, interested, and creative spirit, fully ready for education. However, he required a wheelchair, had only moderate control of his hands, and could not speak words. It wasn't that he couldn't think them; rather, the muscles that fire his vocal chords couldn't coordinate enough to turn sounds into the more nuanced utterances understood by us all as communication.

Faced with those challenges, our family learned about AAC (the device the famed physicist Stephen Hawking used for speech). And doesn't it speak to the arcane nature of AAC that for people to even recognize it, our field usually references its use by a once-in-a-century genius astrophysicist.

As Tom was starting elementary school, in the program we started, he was also progressing with his augmentative communication. I was one of those parents who wanted to program the device, and provide all the support I could for my child. But it just . . . took . . . so . . . long!

Today, 20 years down the road, I better understand how challenging it is to create tech for such a small population. But back then, as an advertising creative director who got to play with the latest boggling technology, it was hard to feel much love for a box that looked like a brick, sounded mechanical, processed at an absurdly slow speed, and showed graphics that didn't elevate expectations of the person using them, but perhaps actually lowered them.

One night at 1:00 a.m., lying in bed having finished hours and hours on the box's clunky interface, knowing the upload would take hours, and hoping the device would not do its typical crash before I woke up, I sat up. And I began thinking.

Sure, I didn't know how to code—and back then I barely knew the difference between RAM and ROM—but in my career, I had certainly seen what tech could create. And I always had a slightly startling innate ability to understand not only the creative problems tech could best solve, but also how to put together seemingly unrelated ideas to create new possibilities and solutions.

In the next few months, I hit the road and met with most of the existing AAC manufacturers. I attended conferences. I went to lectures and met the best presenters at the bar get-togethers to drink and talk more. They were all terrific. But, of course, like most people and companies, they had their own way of doing things. Their perspective was also dominated by current technology, as well a sprinkle of pedagogy. The communication I envisioned was something different; it came from Madison Avenue.

One night, lying in a hotel outside of Minneapolis, thinking of Tom, and still buzzing from all I had listened to, I was stunned as I thought to myself: "Darn. I'm going to leave advertising and invent my own device."

* * *

Blink Twice and our product, The Tango, were introduced in 2007. The Tango looked like a wild, fanciful, oversized alien Tylenol capsule. It was white, silver, and gorgeous. It was designed not only to build sentences, but also relationships.

Assistive technology was large and bulky and mechanical back then; devices opened doors to language but also created so many new barriers. People had told me that the greatest problem in the field was abandonment (for Heaven's sake!). SLPs told me that, despite themselves, they often felt frustrated waiting for people to speak simple things. What a tough, dispiriting problem. But I knew we could change things by leveraging what I knew of mass consumer communication. A great tagline was, "You never get a second chance to make a first impression." Our field never thought of that. But I knew that, to create success, we needed to change the expectations that were created with that first impression.

The Tango's communication structure blended generative synthetic speech with thousands of engaging pre-recorded messages. It brought new life to simple thoughts like greetings, wants, and feedback about things one likes and dislikes, all of which can be reasonably anticipated. And it brought it together in an easy-to-navigate interface.

The Tango embraced the need to learn advanced communication but also the deep human need to share, to have friends, to experience *connection*. Instead of the traditional huge box mounted on a pole, which so often blocked a person's face and expression, the Tango was low-slung, providing a greater chance for visual engagement. The Tango introduced Tango Symbols (now Tobii-Dynavox PCS Persona symbols), which brought a fresh, engaging sensibility to the serious task of communication symbols.

As I tell my son, I can't begin to imagine the challenge of communicating using AAC or the perseverance required to succeed. That being said, it's important to also accept that conversations incorporating AAC can also be difficult for the listener. We live in a world where communication crackles at the speed of electricity, where tone is as important as content. And so, whether fair or not, it's a lot to ask the rest of the world to slow down for AAC. And we need to think through that, too. The Tango was given its name, because it takes two to tango, in this case, the speaker *and* the listener.

The world took notice of the Tango because it was designed not only to help people communicate but to help others look at disabilities, differently. The Tango's DNA was infused with joy and engagement. It provided not only support for nonverbal individuals but also respect and understanding for the needs of the entire communication circle, including the speaker, parents, friends, teachers, and SLPs.

The Tango leveraged an advertising creative executive's understanding that much of what we say *can* be planned, that we can balance our need for generative language with the stuff we constantly repeat. (Seriously, think of your own speech patterns. So much of what we all say, we say over and over, repeating favorite stories, jokes, joys, experiences, and complaints.) Being nonverbal is not a typical condition. So why do we approach nonverbal communication with the same word-by-word sentence building as we do for verbal communicators? Can't there be something better?

One of my great joys over these years was to have shared these insights with some of the field's most remarkable thinkers: Pati King DeBaun, Caroline Musselwhite (read Caroline's story on page 1), Karen Erickson, and Linda Burkhart at the start, and later with Mo Buti, Deanna Wagner, Gretchen Hanser, and Megan Fucci-Wenzel—and to have them so generously help me merge this socially oriented thinking with their knowledge and insight about AAC and language in general. They all became part of Team Tango. And then there was Patrick Brune, who worked at our company, not only helping develop our structure, but also crafting the messaging that the world could best hear and implement. Tango would not have happened without him.

I still remember putting up our very first booth at an AAC conference, Closing The Gap. Instead of the typical dull stock-photos and two-dimensional exhibition spaces that dominated the field back then, we erected a 10 x 25 room, with walls made of white parachute material highlighting a huge image of the Tango and our logo. As we began putting it up, all the other booths took a break, stopped, and watched. Something new was happening.

The Tango announced that the person who used it was cool and playful and had compelling things to share—not simply that the person using it required technology to communicate. The Tango challenged the field to do more, which it has, especially as assistive technology has become so much more in sync with consumer tech. Think of it: back at the, um, turn of the century, going about with an electronic box featuring a grid-based navigational system seemed so odd.

Today, that description pretty much applies to everyone. Thanks, Apple. We owe you one.

* * *

The world embraced not only the Tango, but also the story behind it. My son and I were featured as *ABC World News* People of the Week and then with a smaller group chosen as People of the Year. Tom and I were on the cover of *Exceptional Parent*, as well as in many articles in local media and TV.

Then, another highlight. Tom was an assistant manager of a Little League Team in Greenwich Village. Using his Tango, he would read the line-up each week and play prerecorded cheers and trumpet calls. And, with no tech required, he gave every batter a high-five before they went to the plate.

When his team won the local league championship, they were chosen to be part of the New York Yankees' first Hope Week (Helping Others Persevere and Excel) at Yankee Stadium, which recognized individuals with challenges who went above and beyond in pursuing their dreams. ESPN's *E:60* did a special segment on Tom's day, as they got to meet many Yankees, throw out the first pitch, and high-five players at the end of the game. Tom began a long friendship with the pitcher Joba Chamberlain, and for five years, they celebrated their birthdays together. The press passes from the day and dirt-smeared batting gloves A-Rod gave him as they high-fived still hang in a frame on Tom's wall.

We often hear that we shouldn't call people with disabilities "heroes," that we shouldn't be "inspired" by their pursuit of a life they envision for themselves.

But if we are inspired by baseball players, why not people with disabilities? The world needs stories of individuals who strive. And when challenges are exaggerated due to disabilities, doesn't that effort deserve a spotlight? Be open to that celebration. Share it with others. Let others see the joy in our lives. Build that bridge. Build an audience.

We fight for our children. We fight for inclusion. For resources. For technology. We advocate for the patience that allows our children to shine, or at least to be noticed. But amid all that struggle, we need to celebrate. Children need to feel joy, love, and a warm cuddly embrace so they will learn that it can happen elsewhere.

Creating the Tango was the joy of a lifetime. It brought together the depth of my feelings toward my son and of his world with the enjoyment of a highly intellectual pursuit. AAC is a puzzle that our passionate and committed team worked to solve. We gave our best efforts to bringing a greater awareness of design and engagement to the field, to helping us all think bigger, and to expecting more. And in 2011, it made sense to merge our company, products, and thinking into DynaVox (now Tobii Dynavox). Our work had been extremely rewarding, but it had also been extremely hard. So for me, a sabbatical felt like a good idea. Maybe even retirement. Whatever was next could wait.

* * *

In 2013, after two years enjoying time with my family, the Cerebral Palsy International Research Foundation (CPIRF) contacted me, and I became their CEO. At the time, CPIRF had little recognition outside of the medical profession, no signature consumer events, and no specific initiatives. Okay, I thought: one last dance.

Medical research and implementation are, of course, critical. However, I also saw a chance to run the Foundation as a chance to address a much broader vision, particularly about the unilluminated perceptions others have about the lives of people with CP—and the much broader ways we could help improve those lives.

In my five years at the Foundation, we changed our name to simply the Cerebral Palsy Foundation, which was much more memorable and accessible.

And once again, all I had learned in advertising helped lead me forward. My first initiative was to develop a new marketing campaign: "Just Say Hi." I asked William H. Macy (who had done a movie, *Door To Door*, about Bill Porter, a salesman with CP) to do our first social media spot. Despite his busy schedule, he was more than willing: What a champ he was to be the first one in the pool! And, two years later, we had more than two dozen celebrities sharing our message, including Alex Rodriguez, Gayle King, and John Oliver. I was thrilled—and boggled—when both Tim Cook and Satya Nadella added their voice to our message, addressing the awkward hesitation faced by so many people with disabilities.

"How do you start a conversation with someone who has disabilities? Just Say Hi." Those words were heard by tens of millions in our country. And so many minds opened up to the possibilities of new connection.

That campaign began the Foundation's journey from an organization focused primarily on medical research to one addressing a bigger problem in the world of disabilities: There are many interventions and resources available, but far too often people didn't receive them. Why?

The answer, I felt, was that we needed the magical realism of marketing. We needed a fresher, unexpected way of communicating that put our world's atypical challenges into a more typical context: to make these issues feel immediate, urgent, and relatable and to tap into the universals of the human condition. As I looked at what the Foundation could accomplish, I continually asked myself how we could build a bridge that others would cross.

To do this, the Foundation began creating vibrant new language. We evolved the Just Say Hi campaign to work in the NYC Public Schools. We developed a Design For Disability Competition, where young fashion designers were mentored by some of fashion's top icons—Thom Browne, Anna Sui, and Derek Lam—who worked in tandem with people with disabilities to create accessible fashion. We consulted with Microsoft during the development of the Xbox Adaptive Controller. We had Apple support us as we shared the importance of fitness for people with disabilities. When *Speechless* was launched on ABC as the first-ever show whose main character had disabilities, we provided thoughtful feedback and input. I personally read every script prior to shooting, to help the writers ensure accuracy and to isolate moments of truth. And we built relationships with extraordinary individuals like Zac Anner and Micah Fowler, who helped us gain exposure through social videos that reached tens of millions.

I left the Foundation in early 2019. However, those five years bristled with so many moments that were so fresh within the context of a not-for-profit organization. As you read the list above, you can envision the magic and passion that built deep relationships between the Foundation and so many world-class companies and renowned individuals. Today, the Foundation is one of the leading voices in the field, and another cherished—and unexpected—part of my history.

* * *

However, again, in a world as small as the world of disabilities, wonderful work is also really exhausting work. And after five years, it was time to retire.

Except . . .

Assistive technology and AAC have evolved so much since I entered the field. What once required millions of dollars and huge investment in hardware, manufacturing, and distribution can be built today on innovatively designed software and distributed through one click in the App Store. It's an exciting and rejuvenating time to be creating new tech, especially while watching one's children head toward adulthood and new adventures. Tom is now in college and has his own apartment. My daughter, Taite, is starting her first year at Cornell, interested in both astrophysics and philosophy! My wife is in her own "third act" job, heading the Division of Gynecological Pathology at Memorial Sloan Kettering. Amid all that, I kept hearing the siren call of the newly energetic field that was my first love: augmentative communication.

And so, I created a new AAC app, Talk Suite, released in 2020.

Like any good AAC app, Talk Suite supports the growth of strong generative language; however, it also incorporates the strong social focus of all my work and provides a structure that allows individuals to better plan and manage a more engaging communication approach. It is based on a novel concept: Anticipatory Communication. Think of it . . . So much of what we say we repeat over and over throughout the years: our favorite stories, the things we love, the things we get angry about, our favorite music, teams, and activities. When we return from a vacation, how often do we tell people about it? And how often is that story almost exactly the same? Or, what about the questions during Circle Time in school? The weather, the day of the week, who is present. Those answers may rotate, but they sure don't change. Talk Suite builds that insight into its very fabric so people who rely on AAC can more quickly access and share the things that show their intelligence and ability, as well as the stories and fun that make them unique and interesting. You can see more about anticipatory communication on Talk-Suite.com and on our YouTube channel.

* * *

Just as this chapter began with my son's story, it will end with another one.

Tom loves Broadway. It gives him passion, belief, depth, escape, and joy. It has also given him community. Tom has been embraced by so many actors and producers who find his passion remarkable and affecting. As one of Tom's favorite Broadway people once said to him, "How wonderful! You've found a world where people don't look to see why you're the same. They want to know why you're different."

In 2017, working with his friend, the actor Christopher Hanke, Tom wrote a one-man show titled *It is What it Is.* He then entered NYC'S One Festival competition and won. The prize was the chance to put on a five-night performance at an off-off-Broadway theater.

Watching the show was one of the most powerful experiences of my life. It was the culmination of all the dreams I had that day back in 2004 as I looked at the cover of the Sunday *New York Times Magazine* and saw my son, smiling to the world—his skinned knee showing beneath the tray of his wheelchair—looking somewhat up and off-camera, as if trying to articulate a future absolutely none of us could have begun to imagine. His use of language was also the culmination of the hopes I had when the first Tango came off the production line.

During Tom's 45-minute show, the script of which he had not shared with me in advance, I was able to see the depth at which my son was processing his life and experiences. I also saw the courage with which he was observing *all* that happened to him—the achievements and the difficulties, the highs and lows, the loves and the distances. And I was able to see how well he could communicate it all. There were so many wonderful jokes and lines, such as his opening, "I see you're staring at me. Don't feel awkward. I'm the only one on the stage."

Tom's show was about meeting girlfriends and his take on each of them. I was confused, as that hadn't really been the case in his life. But then, about two-thirds in, Tom shattered his narrative. In an astonishing and devastating twist, the narrative turned to the reality: that he made all those people up. He admits to loneliness, yet also to a belief that he will one day indeed find someone. It is stunning moment, for it is the human experience, the comingling of challenge and hope, that daunting, ever-beating desire we all share: to be understood.

Tom's show breaks your heart, and then puts it back together. His message, coming through his iPad, could not have been louder. And, through more than a few tears, I could not have been prouder.

Recommendations

I have always thought that my role, whether for my son, my family, my career, or my life, has been to open doors through which others can go: to set a stage, so to speak. Once someone has gone there, success or failure is up to them.

In doing so, it is such a joy to see what happens as *others* go into those rooms, to see ideas nurtured, grown, changed, sometimes embraced, sometimes rejected, but always evolved in unexpected ways. In that way, I hope I have done my part to leave things better than when I came along. And I don't think there is a better definition of purpose in life.

At every crossroads, I have paused to set my expectations. And then, I have trusted in the unexpected.

Be open to that. Embrace it. Build on it. Joy awaits.

My Community

Watch my interview with Mai Ling Chan on Cognixion's What's New? What's Next? in AAC:

Ways to Connect with Me

Email: richarde@talk-suite.com

To learn more about Talk Suite: www.Talk-Suite.com

Facebook: http://bit.ly/TS-FBook

Richard Ellenson has spent two decades sharing a vibrant and innovative voice in the disabilities space. He worked with some of the field's top speech professionals to create the influential AAC device, the Tango, and later created the AAC app, Talk Suite Pro. He has received two National Institute of Health (NIH) grants, sat on NIH advisory councils for both the National Institute on Deafness and Other Communication Disorders (NIDCD) and the National Center for Medical Rehabilitation Research (NCMRR), and given keynote addresses on three continents. Prior to his work in the disability space, Richard was an advertising executive who created memorable campaigns for brands such as American Express, Remy Martin, and HBO. Richard is the father of a magnificent 23-year-old, Thomas, who has cerebral palsy.

Together, they have been featured as *ABC World News People of the Year*, in a *New York Times Sunday Magazine* cover story, and on many local news segments, as well as a feature segment on ESPN's *E:60*.

PrAACtical Adventures: An Introvert's Journey into Public Spaces

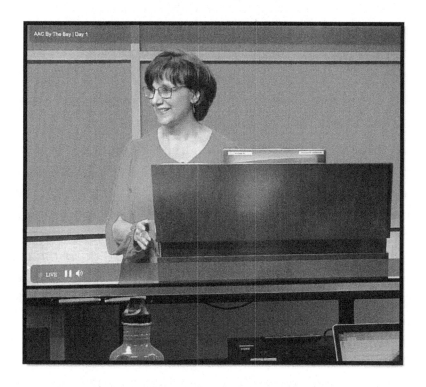

Carole Zangari, PhD, CCC-SLP

* * *

In our society, growing older is not something most people look forward to. Time and gravity take a toll and their impact can be most unwelcome. It is true that our bodies become less reliable, and, I believe American society, in general, holds deeply negative views of aging, but that's only part of the story. In my experience, something wonderful happens as you age: you worry less about what others think and you gain confidence in your own vision, just at the time when experience allows you to be more effective in solving problems and overcoming hurdles. There is power in that combination, and it's what led me to the creation of one of the world's most popular augmentative and alternative communication (AAC) websites, PrAACtical AAC.

My AAC story began some decades ago. It's hard to pinpoint where my interest in alternative ways of communicating really began, but I think Mr. Stefanik played a role in it.

In the early 1970s, I was too young to be left at home alone all summer while my parents were working. I had little interest in summer camp and was too young for a work permit. My mom's solution was to take me to work with her and it shaped the rest of my life. I got an alarm clock for my 12th birthday and set it every morning for 5:45 a.m. so I could go with her to a skilled nursing facility where she was a well-respected charge nurse. I was too young to be a candy striper so the administrators just looked the other way, and I found ways to make myself useful. One of my jobs was to deliver mail to the residents. My favorite part was going to the second floor, especially on the days when Mr. Stefanik got mail from overseas, and I saved that chore for last.

In those days, airmail envelopes were exotic things. The thin paper envelopes with their red, white, and blue borders promised a peek into countries I'd only read about in schoolbooks and National Geographic magazines. Mr.

Stefanik, a resident who kept to himself and rarely came out of his room, was the only one I knew who received these foreign treasures, and I was determined to share in his bounty. He had suffered a stroke, was densely hemiplegic, and had great difficulty expressing himself. Although I didn't know it then, he had profound apraxia of speech. Mr. Stefanik clearly understood everything he heard and read, but his attempts to speak were sidelined by endless groping for the sounds he was looking for and this brought him shame and despair. He was a persistent communicator, though, and through one-armed gestures, pantomime, and objects in the environment, he usually found a way to get his point across.

I had so many questions for him. Why was he getting letters from far away with beautiful stamps that I didn't recognize? Who was writing to him and why? What did they say? Most of the time, the letters were in languages I didn't understand, so it was up to Mr. Stefanik—incredibly limited in writing and speaking ability—to explain it all to me. And explain he did. In bits and pieces, I learned that he had been a performer in his younger days and had traveled throughout Europe as a high-wire walker. He scaled buildings, walked atop bridges, performed in circuses, and traversed ravines in Hungary, Serbia, and Romania. Over months, I learned that he had served in the army, ran away to pursue his dreams of being a performer, found love and lost it, and escaped to a new continent to start life anew. My adolescent brain was mesmerized.

And so, it seemed natural to me that communication could happen not just in words, but also by pointing to stamps and magazine pictures, gesturing, grunting, showing objects, whistling, and pantomiming. Mr. Stefanik taught me about patience (he grunted and growled if I tried to rush him) and persistence (he'd bang his quad cane on the floor if I gave up trying to understand him), but mostly he taught me this: everyone communicates, and their stories are worth listening to.

When Matthew, a 7-year-old boy with a severe head injury, was admitted to the nursing home (as a favor from the director of nursing, who was the boy's neighbor and my mom's friend), the nursing staff made me a very informal part of his care team. As a result of my participation, I learned to perform passive range of motion activities and cognitive stimulation before I hit puberty and knew all about Berta and Karel Bobath—and their clinical treatment approach for adults with stroke and children with cerebral palsy—before I was old enough to drive. In the weeks and months of coma recovery, Matthew's alertness and skills improved, and my role morphed into one of friend and translator. Communicating in alternative ways was a major part of our journey together.

Little did I know that this area of communication, which I had grown to love, was emerging as an area of focus at the same time. Eventually, as an undergraduate speech-language pathologist (SLP) student at the University of Pittsburgh, I took courses in nonverbal communication and learned about Blissymbolics, a semantic graphical language, and voice output communication aids (VOCAs) in my graduate course in cerebral palsy. When I had the opportunity to complete clinical rotations with people who had little or no functional speech, I felt like I had come home. I was on cloud nine.

My very first SLP job, serving a caseload of adults who had severe challenging behavior and intellectual disabilities, brought me back to reality. I loved the work, often arriving early and staying late. The shadow side to that experience was that I often felt unprepared and incompetent. When you try to administer a formal test and a 325-pound woman pins you to the wall, it makes you realize how much you have to learn about being a good therapist.

Years later, when I earned my PhD and was teaching AAC classes at Purdue University, those experiences influenced the way I designed the coursework and clinical experiences. Theory and research are important touchstones, but unless you know a little something about the practicalities of good therapy, you'll never get to apply them. I guess I was practical even before I developed PrAACtical AAC.

I spent my career in academia, teaching AAC classes, working with student clinicians, directing dissertations, and running a number of different AAC programs. As in many workplaces, higher education is often weighed down in bureaucracy and has challenges familiar to many professions. While I have been fortunate to work with many colleagues who are supportive and collaborative, I've also had experiences with administrators who wielded their power in unhelpful ways.

We've all been buried in paperwork and done enough busy work to make our eyes glaze over. Many of us have had experiences with people who micromanage us, rules that don't make sense, and bosses who think intimidation is an effective approach to leadership. On the good days, we rise above the nonsense; and on the bad days, we wallow in it. And on the very bad days, we grit our teeth, and tell ourselves, "there has to be a better way."

PrAACtical AAC was born on one of those dark days. I had just gone toe-to-toe with an administrator who was unhappy that I used an old form to complete the hiring process for someone in our AAC preschool. We did the advertising according to specifications, held the interviews with all the right people, got feedback from the interviewing committee, and completed all of the background checks. We were ready to hire, but the form I had given the interviewers to rate each applicant had been replaced with an updated one. Even though the people in charge had never informed us of that change, they judged our search and hiring process to be invalid. I proposed a simple solution: each interviewer could copy their ratings and comments from the old form to the new one. Problem solved! Or maybe not. The administration's solution was different: scrap the whole process and start over. I wanted to scream, cry, and throw myself to the ground. It was all I could do not to quit.

When things are very bad, a tried-and-true strategy is to vent to a friend. As luck would have it, the friend and colleague to whom I turned was Robin Parker. Coincidentally, Robin was also experiencing frustrations in her work life at that time, so we shared our woes, gnashed our teeth, ordered appetizers, and polished off a nice bottle of wine.

At the end of our commiserating, we reached two significant conclusions and one important decision. Our conclusions? First, the points of aggravation and frustration were likely to continue. Secondly, for the sake of our sanity, we needed to do something where we were in control of the process and could make our own decisions without any chain of approval. Our important decision? It was time to do an AAC project together outside of our workspace. We decided to build our own little happy place and we did.

For the next many months, we met at each other's homes and in parks. We took long walks and sat staring at the ocean. We called each other a few times a day, we learned new things, and we stepped out of our comfort zone. We lived and breathed PrAACtical AAC. We had plenty of missteps and failures along the way, lots of fatigue, and self-doubt, and we had our share of cringe-worthy moments. But what we both realized is this: the worst day of failing in your own dream space is better than the best day of working in someone else's vision.

This was ours. PrAACtical AAC would rise or fall on its merits, and that was okay with us. It was invigorating to have that sort of control, and despite the setbacks, we found joy in the journey.

"The soul's joy lies in doing."[6] - Percy Bysshe Shelley

In 2011, we launched the first version of the PrAACtical AAC website.

Why did two middle-aged, not-so-tech-savvy, fairly introverted professors decide to make their AAC musings public? Why not do something less stressful and more in line with our comfort zone and skillset? Why take the risk of such a public failure? Truthfully, it was, once again, because we were fed up. We were really fed up.

We were fed up with watching kids go to kindergarten without a robust form of communication. We were fed up with

---

[6] https://www.brainyquote.com/quotes/percy_bysshe_shelley_120950

Individualized Education Programs (IEPs) that vastly underestimated students' potential. We were fed up with meeting teenagers who were never given access to a language system they could utilize and build on. We were fed up with talking to desperate parents who were begging for help. We were fed up with clinicians who were not providing adequate services, and we were fed up with systems that perpetuated poor service delivery. So, we started a blog.

Blogs were new at that time and much disparaged in academic circles. No serious scholar would write a blog, we were told, "It will hurt your career." "You're already at a teaching university." They said, "Shouldn't you focus on things that can bolster your reputation and enhance your CV?" The implications were clear: *This is beneath you.*

To us, it didn't feel that way at all.

We decided to write the blog that we wish had been around when we were first starting out. One with quality content that educated people on the *why* and also helped them with the *how*. We had no idea how to create a blog or use social media, and we had no budget for any sort of help, but we weren't going to let that stop us.

Over time, we built PrAACtical AAC into a valuable resource that exceeded our original expectations. We found joy in the process.

Tragically, though, Robin succumbed to cancer in 2014. PrAACtical AAC continued to be a happy place for her throughout her illness, and it has been my honor to continue it in the six years since her passing.

These last few years, PrAACtical AAC has grown and evolved. It has moved to new platforms, used new designs, and seen some features flourish while others wither away. It has readers in 229 regions across the globe and has had more than a million page views each year since 2015. It is used in graduate-level courses by respected AAC instructors and is frequently cited by AAC presenters at state and national conferences. Most importantly, it has elevated the AAC knowledge base of families and AAC practitioners and given several of them a platform from which to share their own work. PrAACtical AAC is now more than a website. It is a community.

Throughout my career, one of my guiding precepts has been this old adage: *To whom much is given, much is expected.* I tend not to think much about what I get in return so the opportunity to reflect on that has been interesting.

Creating and managing PrAACtical AAC has been a catalyst for growth in several ways. On a personal level, it has helped me become more disciplined. We started out publishing new posts each day, and while we now only publish a few times a week, it still requires a commitment to the routine of creating and publishing a lot of content on a regular basis.

Another gift that came through PrAACtical AAC was a greater tolerance for imperfection. My heart wants to spend an hour on every paragraph to get it *just right*, but after more than 2,500 posts, I've learned that sometimes "good enough" is better than "perfection."

Financial gain was never the vision for PrAACtical AAC, although we did explore options to cover the expenses. Robin and I had many, many discussions about the possibility of monetizing the site to offset some of the costs of development, security, and hosting. I continue to get offers for advertising and affiliate marketing, and suggestions to develop a section accessible through a paywall. While there is some appeal to that, it pales in comparison to the satisfaction of knowing that the site is free of obligation to advertisers or paid subscribers. The field of AAC faces enough hurdles without erecting additional barriers to access high-quality information.

There have been countless other benefits of my journey with PrAACtical AAC, as well, not the least of which, are the many wonderful families, AAC users, and professionals who I have met through this platform. The greatest gift, however, is that it has provided me with an ongoing connection to Robin, who was taken from us far too soon.

Recommendations

Here are a few recommendations I have for those of you looking to grow and expand your AAC skills and offerings.

1. **Trust yourself.** You didn't get to this place by accident. Your instincts, experiences, talents, and values are hidden assets that brought you here. They will be far better guides than the message in any book, presentation, podcast, or website.

2. **Know when "good enough" is good enough.** I was once brought into a situation where there was disagreement among IEP team members about how to best help a student with AAC needs. Jaime had stalled out on his goal to make relevant comments in his interactions with adults and peers with 80% in three consecutive sessions. He started off strong but in the

final quarter of the academic year, his performance bounced around between 70% and 85%. One day, he'd get 76%, and the next day, he'd get 88%, and then back to 79%. Some team members thought they should keep working on that goal until Jaime consistently was above 80%. Others thought an average of 80% was good enough. Getting to consistency meant that Jaime would be working on this goal for another three to six months, and that meant that we'd be postponing his opportunity to develop other sorts of language skills. Consistency is important in learning to use the toilet or cross the street, but making a relevant comment with 80% accuracy? Not so much. The opportunity costs were just too great.

Sometimes, actually MANY times, "good enough" is good enough. Just like the saying, *Perfection is the enemy of the good.*

3. **Be prepared to tear down things that you build.** Sometimes things that you spend a lot of time on, and really believe in, don't work. My grandfather taught me that pruning is the key to healthy growth, and while I mourned for the weaker lettuce seedlings that went into the compost pile, I came to see the wisdom at harvest time.

4. **Be original.** Don't be a variation on a theme. Instead, develop an original idea or an original approach to a common problem. Does the world really need another set of pictures or core board or grid display AAC app? I'm not sure, but even if we do, the real fun comes in finding your own idea and helping it blossom. Bringing

your unique solution to a problem, need, or opportunity creates much joy.

5. **Give it your all.** No matter how good the idea is, or how solid the plan is, there is no substitute for hard work.

Communication is every person's birthright, and it is intolerable that some people with disabilities are prevented from accessing robust AAC tools, supports, and services. Our response to communicative inequity and injustice has the power to change lives. Is there a greater feeling than to see someone overcome those barriers and live the life they choose?

In a perfect world, we'd each have the resources we need to pursue the intersection of our passion and our purpose. But where most of us live, the time, money, energy, and institutional support needed for our projects to take wing are in short supply.

Here is my wish for you as you put some wind beneath those wings—I wish that you stay true to yourself, even when you are tempted by *shiny things* and especially when you doubt yourself. Avoid getting constantly distracted by new and exciting things and chasing project after project without clarity. Instead, stay focused on your goal and follow-through with your short and long-term strategies.

Learn to take failure for what it is: a learning experience. Your project may fail, but that doesn't make you a failure.

And I hope that you find your stride in whatever path you choose, and along with it, a congenial companion or community to share in your journey.

My Community

Watch my interview with Mai Ling Chan on Cognixion's What's New? What's Next? in AAC:

Ways to Connect with Me

www.PrAACticalAAC.org

Twitter: @PrAACticalAAC

Instagram: @PrAACticalAAC

LinkedIn: https://bit.ly/CZatLinkedIn

Facebook: www.facebook.com/PrAACticalAAC

Pinterest: www.pinterest.com/aacandat

Dr. Carole Zangari is a professor in the Speech-Language Pathology department at Nova Southeastern University and serves as the executive director of the Broward satellite of the

University of Miami-Nova Southeastern University Center for Autism and Related Disabilities (UM-NSU CARD). Dr. Zangari is also the owner and author of www.PrAACticalAAC.org, co-editor of *Practically Speaking Language, Literacy, and Academic Development for Students with AAC Needs* and coauthor of *TELL ME: AAC in the Preschool Classroom* and *TELL ME Más.*

Getting through Life's Puddles

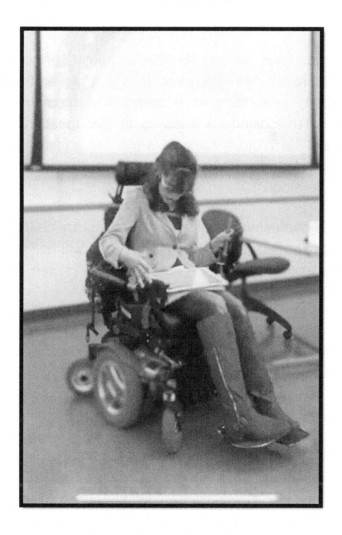

Lydia Dawley, BS

"Every path has puddles. They are just puddles. You'll get through them."

- Grandma Dawley

* * *

I'm on the floor in my brother's house on the most uncomfortable air mattress ever. It is 4 a.m., and I haven't slept yet. My eyes sting from crying. My throat hurts from screaming. I'm looking for answers to the questions, "Why? Why today? Why did it happen when my and my brother's lives were just starting?" This. Is. Definitely. Worse. Than. Not. Being. Understood.

That was a confusing and very dark start to my chapter. But I got you hooked, so ha ha! Don't worry, you will find out about the darkest days of my life later. For now, let me introduce myself properly.

My name is Lydia. I'm a college graduate. I love food. I love to watch *Ellen* EVERY SINGLE DAY! I don't go to bed until 2 a.m., (not even kidding you, it's 1:39 a.m. as I type this). My absolute favorite TV show is *New Girl*. I don't know why, but I don't care for movies. I love music, and I can listen to hip-hop music and country music all day, and I love to dance! I ABSOLUTELY HATE LIVE CHICKENS because I think they are little devils just plotting their revenge. I'm afraid of taxidermy animals. Don't ask me why because I have no idea. I have an older brother, Zach, and I grew up on a farm. I used to show my dog, horse, goats, and sheep at my county's fair. I ran for my county's fair queen and won, so I advanced to compete for the Iowa State Fair Queen, and I was titled Miss Personality Plus. My dad taught me how to drive horses, and I rode horses, too. I was in individual and large group speech competitions and went to state and all-state competitions for both of them. What else do you need to know about me? Oh yes, I forgot to tell you, I have mixed cerebral palsy.

I was born on August 22, 1996, and my birth caused a lot of havoc, but I think it should have warned my parents that I was going to be a fighter. I was positioned bottom-first instead of head-first inside my mom, so the doctors had to apply pressure to my mom's belly to manually turn me while I was still inside her womb. I was born a week later, but I wasn't breathing at all because my umbilical cord was around my neck not once, not twice, but three times. The doctors, nurses, and respiratory therapists worked on me for 17 minutes to bring me back to life. That's how I got cerebral palsy (CP). During the time while I wasn't breathing—well—I was dead. Parts of my brain were not getting oxygen and became damaged. As a result, I have mixed type cerebral palsy, which means I have two different types. I have spastic CP, which makes my muscles very tight and hard for me to stretch out my arms, legs, and fingers. The other type I have is athetoid, which is characterized by uncontrolled movements. When I go to pick something up, my hand will jerk in different directions and it will take me several attempts sometimes to hit my target. I can't walk without assistance from someone, so I use a wheelchair. I talk with an alternative and augmentative communication (AAC) device sometimes, but my family and close friends can understand my verbal speech.

I had to learn how to read at an early age so I could let people know what I needed and what I was thinking. Believe me, I had a lot of thoughts that I wanted to get out. My preschool teacher told my parents, "There is something in this girl's head, and it's called brains." She encouraged my parents to mainstream my education. My preschool teacher also taught me sign language, but it's not American Sign Language like everyone uses because I couldn't manipulate my hands correctly, so she taught me to create the sign I could do that was closest to the target sign—and go with it. She taught me I had to learn how to communicate in non-traditional ways so I could be in a regular classroom, to make friends, and to just get along in life. With her help, I learned to spell words with my hands in the air and had a printed and laminated copy of words that I used to communicate with friends.

This was just the beginning of my journey. Ultimately, I chose to study communication sciences and disorders, at the University of Wisconsin in Whitewater, Wisconsin. This caused a lot of questions and doubts in the department like— "How could a *nonverbal* person teach another person to talk?" But I was determined to break that glass ceiling, so I spent hours and hours studying and researching techniques to be able to personally demonstrate to people how to place their mouth to say a word. I always felt the need to be ready and on my toes 24/7. I couldn't help worrying that if my professors saw me off my A-game, then they would probably doubt me more, and this would negatively affect my ability to complete the program. It was exhausting.

They say that going to college will change your life. You will meet your life-long friends and you have experiences you won't forget. That may be true. I have met my nerdy friends, and I guess I will keep them around. I also think I had a *normal* college experience. I had to hire and fire my own caregivers. Yes, I have fired a caregiver, someone who talked baby talk to me and just couldn't see past my disability. One day, I took my laundry cart to Walmart with my wheelchair because I needed a microwave, and I didn't want to wait until my parents visited to get one. My wheelchair broke down on my way home from class, and my iPad's battery died, so I flagged down a girl to help me. Because she didn't know what I was trying to tell her, she called the campus police. Luckily, the University of Wisconsin-Whitewater has a lot of students in wheelchairs. So, the police were familiar with trying to figure out these issues. They found my override switch and got my wheelchair going. I was feeling pretty proud that I had managed my problem on my own without my parents! I thought I had this college thing down.

Going to college changed my life, but I don't think people meant going to college will change your life 360 degrees. My life did a 360-degree turn, and never stopped turning!

Remember how I started this chapter? Let's go back to that moment of being on the most uncomfortable mattress ever on the floor of my brother's house.

It was Sunday, November 5, 2017. I was in my junior year of college and found out my mom had been trying to reach me. My cousin was already at my apartment waiting to bring me home—my dad was in the hospital. I jumped in the car with my cousin, not really knowing what was happening. It took us five hours to get home, and it was the longest five hours of my life.

"Dad and Zach were chasing cattle. Dad had a heart attack. Zach tried to save him, but it was too late. I'm so sorry honey. Dad passed," my mom said when we arrived.

Those words still sting today. I can still picture that night losing my voice as I screamed, "NO!" until my voice became hoarse. My mom sat and rocked me, with Zach hugging my waist. I didn't sleep for a week, and it was all a blur. Three days after my dad's funeral, I returned to school at Whitewater, three and a half hours away from my family. But I was pretty proud of myself because I did my homework while I was gone, not to mention everything else was also on time.

Dealing with grief, going to class, having homework, having to prove you were worthy of being in a challenging major, managing your caregiver, and balancing your mental health was pretty hard. I secretly got mad when people said they skipped class because they were tired. I thought to myself, "I wish I could skip because I wasn't really here mentally either."

Dreaming about my dad nowadays is still so weird, and it totally messes with my head the rest of the day. When I wake up, I have to remind myself that dad is not here. I remember in the spring semester following his passing, I was in neurology. It was the night before I was studying for the exam the next day, I went to bed, and I had a dream about my dad. When I woke up, I was so confused then I started crying because I realized that it was a dream. I was so off of my game. I went to my exam, everything that I studied was completely gone, so I just guessed every answer.

I eventually graduated from University of Wisconsin, Whitewater with my Bachelor of Science in Liberal Studies with special interest in Communication Sciences and Disorders. I had to change my major as it was hard to focus on school and be on my A-game after my dad passed away, but thankfully, my past courses could count toward my new major. I had no idea what I was going to do as a career because I couldn't be a Speech-Language Pathologist without my bachelor's in communicative disorders.

Then, in March 2020, I had to go back home because of the coronavirus pandemic, which completely stopped my independent life. What do you do when you are home, and finishing your undergraduate degree online? I don't know about other people, but I created my own consulting business!

In April 2020, I applied for an LLC for my new business, Click. Speak. Connect. I called my friend to create a logo, texted my college friend to ask to join me, and on June 8th, I saw my first client— which people said I couldn't do.

I want to help AAC users feel free and engaged in their own communication. I have seen so much progress in my clients in just the four months I have been working with them. I have a client who has a hard time sitting still for a long period of time, but when I meet with her, she is able to sit for a whole hour. I'm so proud of her and each one of my clients. I really feel like I am making a difference. I can see it in the excitement on their faces and in their communication. They are gaining confidence and now they feel comfortable communicating. It's amazing for all of us!

Also, in 2020, we started a Kickstarter campaign. It aims to raise money to help cover the cost of production of the NadPen, a new stylus we plan to start selling in the summer of 2021.

I always needed to make my own styluses. Because of my cerebral palsy, I press down so hard that I tear off the rubber ends of many styluses. First it was tin foil on the end of the stylus, then it was a piece of a sock, and then I used conductive tape on the end of the stylus with two pencils duct taped together.

I had always been told to sell my styluses to others because I wasn't the only one who had a hard time finding a stylus that worked. In May 2017, I started to sell my styluses. It was super hard, and I would have my friends and my mom make them and mail them. We couldn't keep up with demand, and I had to stop selling them.

In October 2020, I was speaking to a school district in California, and I got a message from a speech-language pathology assistant who was interested in creating a prototype of my stylus. It has been a lot of fun and hard work going back and forth with our ideas.

We call this stylus NadPen because N.A.D. are my dad's initials and stand for Nathan Author Dawley. For some reason, farmers, like my dad, always carry a pen in the front pockets of their shirts. If anyone needed a pen, my dad would grab his pen and say, "You can use mine."

To offset the costs of production for the stylus, we launched the Kickstarter campaign at the end of December 2020, and raised $10,456 by February 2021. We are so thankful for everyone who donated to the campaign, and we are working with a manufacturing company to start selling.

For many years, my dad encouraged me, saying, "You have to do this for all of the people who told you no, Lyddie."

Now I can say, "See dad, your Lyddie did it! I hope you are so proud!"

My Inspiration

I always had people who doubted me because of my disability. In middle school, I was placed in special education because some of the teachers did not want me in their classroom. They thought I was too distracting. My parents always told me that I needed to work my butt off to get where I wanted to go in life. I began taking charge of my communication devices and education. I bet some of my teachers and therapists wanted to pull their hair out because I sometimes told them that I didn't like their ideas. Other times, I would straight up tell them I didn't like the device they chose for me to try. It made me realize that I can direct my life toward success.

That is the main reason why I started Click. Speak. Connect. I want to show kids with disabilities that they can tell their parents, educators, or therapists when they don't like something. I'm not saying they need to kick their kindergarten aide to get their point across like I did, but children need to learn independence and autonomy. We as educators need to teach decision-making and communicating our feelings way before we teach daily activities. To have total independence, we need to be able to share our opinions and be confident while doing so.

Another inspiration for starting Click. Speak. Connect. are my parents. They let me take charge of my life, and they believed in me since day one. I have seen parents of children with disabilities who took their children to the same therapies as me, turn into "helicopter parents" who do everything for their child. My parents learned early on that I was stubborn. I had a Rifton walker that I would tear around in, and I would get so frustrated with my parents because they couldn't understand what I was saying, so I would ram my walker into them to get them to really concentrate on my speech. I wouldn't be where I am today if it wasn't for my parents letting me learn to self-advocate. That's another reason why I wanted to open Click. Speak. Connect— because I want to work with parents and help them realize that their kids will be alright if they don't do everything for them and, instead, encourage self-advocacy.

Recommendations

1. If something doesn't work today, it doesn't mean that it will never work!

2. Nonverbal people have things to say, but our bodies don't let us.

3. People with disabilities do not want sympathy. We want friendships and to be given a chance to live a life like everyone else. We didn't choose this life, but since we were given the challenge, we sometimes have to count on others.

My favorite person, my grandma Dawley, who loved to read till her last day on earth, would recite these inspirational quotes from various people to me:

"Sister, every path has a few puddles. They are just puddles. You'll get through them."

"Don't wait for the perfect moment. Take the moment and make it perfect."

"Somewhere out there, your name is being called to something very special. Listen to the call that gives you the fullness of life and follow it wherever it might lead you."

"You must make the choice—to take a chance—if you want to make a change."

"People will forget what you say, people will forget what you did, but people will never forget how you make them feel."

"As you move on with your life, you can follow someone else's script, try to make choices that will make other people happy, avoid discomfort, do what is expected, and copy the status quo. Or you can look at all that you have accomplished and use it as fuel to venture forth and write your own story."

My Community

Watch my interview with Mai Ling Chan on Cognixion's What's New? What's Next? in AAC:

Ways to Connect with Me

www.clickspeakconnect.com

Facebook: @clickspeakconnect

Instagram: @click.speak.connect

Lydia Dawley is from Decorah, Iowa, and recently graduated from the University of Wisconsin in Whitewater with a bachelor of science. She is the chief executive officer and founder of Click. Speak. Connect. where she consults with speech-language pathologists, teachers, parents, and clients on access methods, faster access, and device experiences to help with learning new apps and language skills related to AAC.

Creating Language Out of Necessity

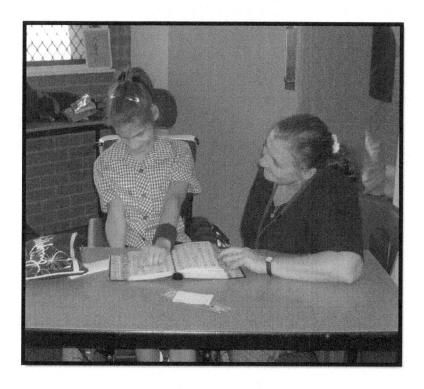

Gayle Porter, SLP

* * *

I never intended to be a product developer. I see myself as a clinical speech-language pathologist and an AAC educator. The Pragmatic Organisation Dynamic Display (PODD) communication system I developed as a commercial resource was a side effect of that work. Sometimes you just have to be prepared to go where life takes you.

As I reflect on my professional journey, I realise how fortunate I was in the places I was employed, the people I worked with, and the experiences gained early in my career. As a new graduate speech pathologist, I was excited to get a job, any job.

My luck was to get a position in 1982 with a very dynamic, forward-thinking team at a rural centre for children and adults with physical disabilities. On my first day, the manager gave me an article on the conductive education concept of "holistic intervention" and the "integrated day" and informed me that at this centre, "She who teaches, toilets."

The children's learning was not to be segmented by professional discipline. Professionals needed to interact with the child as a complete person. Therapists at this centre did not take clients off into their separate clinic rooms to "do therapy." Instead, we were scheduled into the early childhood and school classrooms for whole mornings or afternoons and expected to implement all daily routine, social, and academic activities. This required therapists and teachers to both teach and learn across disciplines to apply the recommended strategies and techniques within the genuine mess of classroom life.

This style of intervention meant that the actual usefulness, or not, of my recommended AAC strategies was continuously *in my face*. It stimulated the type of questions that have proven useful throughout my career: Why are we doing this? What is the purpose of this? Does it make a difference to the person's life? What's missing?

When I transferred to a centre in Metropolitan Melbourne (Australia) I brought these questions with me. This centre had a much larger population of adults who required AAC services, in addition to early childhood and school-age classrooms. The existing model of service delivery for a speech pathologist in the adult services was individual speech pathology sessions (in my office) and leading a few communication-focused group programs with the day centre staff.

After leading the existing communication board users and signing groups for some time, I became frustrated that my clients seemed to be developing a lot of AAC skills that I did not see being used at other times. I proposed to my manager that, instead of running communication focused groups, I would join other existing group activities to focus on problem solving and teaching other staff and clients how AAC can be used for genuine purposes throughout the day. This was perhaps my first conscious foray into what we would now call a more systemic approach to AAC intervention, with a focus on developing an accessible communication community. It had mixed results.

One of the group activities I joined was the video group. We had a great year with people using AAC to actively contribute concepts and ideas to the script and production. The day centre staff was extremely enthusiastic about the process, and everyone applauded the resulting video.

At the end of the first year, I thought that the staff had developed sufficient skills to use AAC in this context without my continuous presence, so I changed to a different group the following year. However, my bubble burst when a staff member told me, "We missed you in video group today. I felt really guilty that we didn't use AAC."

I was disappointed to say the least. It is not enough to enable interaction using AAC only when I am there. As a speech pathologist, I can be present for so little of a person's life. In moments like these, it is really easy to give up and to ask yourself, "What is the point?"

Perseverance (stubbornness), a belief in the possibilities of AAC and the lyrics from the musical Oliver—"I'm reviewing the situation . . . I think I'd better think it out again"[7]—are helpful at times like these. Let's review the situation: they may not have applied what I thought I had taught, but at least they recognized that the absence of AAC was a problem. After all, recognizing the need for change is the first step toward creating cultural change.

For the remainder of the 1980s, I continued working with a range of people who use AAC in a variety of services, including early childhood, school, adult day centre, sheltered workshops, and accommodation units. Working in the community and problem solving with adults who use AAC was very instructive for my future work. I was inspired by some of my client's determination to be heard and engaged. They used AAC to get out there and live their lives, and AAC enabled them to achieve their goals.

The advent of speech-generating devices brought an additional dimension to the possibilities and problems that

---

[7] DeTurk, Scott. *The Musical Adventures of Oliver Twist*: Adapted from the Classic Novel by Charles Dickens. Englewood, Colo.: Pioneer Drama Service, 1999.

needed to be solved. Successes, failures, and frustrations developed my understanding to respond to these fundamental questions: Why are we doing this? What is the purpose of this? Does it make a difference to the person's life? What's missing?

During this period, there was also an increase in the availability of AAC literature. The *Augmentative and Alternative Communication* journal began publication in 1985. I loved reading editorials and articles aimed at clarifying the purpose of AAC and evaluating its significance for people who have complex communication needs. I couldn't get enough of life stories shared by people who use AAC, because they deepened my understanding. A few articles, in particular, stimulated my thinking, including Janice Light's 1989 definition of communication competence and a series of three articles from Light, Collier, and Parnes (1985 a, b, & c) that shared their research on communication modes, functions, and discourse in interactions between children who use AAC and their primary caregivers. Together, with some of my Australian AAC colleagues, we witnessed a renaissance of thought and discussion around the pragmatic use of AAC. I sought out any writings and stories shared by people who use AAC for information about their real life uses, challenges, and suggestions. It became clear to me that the pragmatic use of AAC was the central component for meaningful outcomes.

To spend more time with my son, I asked to work part-time after maternity leave. To accommodate this request, in 1990 my caseload shifted to focus on early intervention services with children who had physical disabilities ages zero to six years old. This early childhood service offered families a choice of home visits or a group program based on the principles of conductive education. Later on, speech pathology services to children in mainstream schools were added to my caseload.

The now famous PODD communication system was developed over the next 17 years as a side effect of clinical problem solving and the development of individual AAC systems for these children and their families. I would like to say there was a comprehensive plan to develop the PODD system, but my plans were more focused on achieving good outcomes for the individual children, families, and their communication partners into the future.

A crucial element in effective problem solving, I have found, is cognitive clarity about the desirable, long-term outcomes. When Alice in Wonderland asked the Cheshire cat, "Would you tell me, please, which way I ought to go from here?" he responded, "That depends a good deal on where you want to get to."[8] When I began developing the PODD system I did not have a communication system as a destination, but I brought with me all the questions, ideas, and experiences gained in interacting with adults who use AAC to this task. Working with young children and their families added another question: How do we stimulate a developmental process and help parents with the knowledge, judgement, and skills to raise their children in a way that leads to the eventual destination?"

Again, I was fortunate to find myself working with a like-minded trans-disciplinary team of dynamic, passionate, progressive professionals. Notably, this team included speech

---

[8] Carroll, Lewis. *Alice's Adventures in Wonderland*. New York: Macmillan, 1920

pathologists Jann Kirkland (B. App. Sc, speech pathology) and Louise Dunne (B. App. Sc, speech pathology), occupational therapists Claire Cotter (B. App. Sc, OT) and Yvette Laurel (B. App. Sc, OT), and physiotherapist Lynn Carter (Dip. of physiotherapy). We all had experience interacting with adults who had physical disabilities and shared a long-term perspective on the joys and challenges of AAC. Together we spent many hours discussing the ideas and concepts that ultimately formed the founding principles for the PODD communication system.

This general aim for AAC provided a vision to guide dynamic assessment and intervention and the criteria for evaluating outcomes: For the person to meet his/her varied communication requirements as intelligibly, specifically, efficiently, independently, and in as socially valued a manner as possible to understand others and to be understood.

A pivotal moment for me in the development of the PODD system came while attending a workshop by Carol Goossens on the topic of engineering the environment for aided language stimulation in 1992 or 1993. As she spoke about the need to engineer the environment to model aided language, Jann Kirkland and I turned to each other and said "DA!" This was because as soon as she said it, the need was so obvious. Why hadn't we thought of engineering the environment? It was a real aha moment.

Aided Language Stimulation, by Goossens, Crain, and Elder, became my favourite book, reading and re-reading until the cover disintegrated. As I read the book, I frantically began making aided language displays for every activity in our group. Fortunately, before I gave everybody on the team a nervous breakdown, Jann reminded me, "Carol Goossens said it took her 10 years!"

The fact that the intervention model we used for group programs was a transdisciplinary team implementing principles of conductive education made us realize a critical factor. We needed more than daily routine or play-based activity displays engineered into our physical environment. For example, we needed more general vocabulary when the children were moving from place to place between activities. Parental questions and feedback also highlighted the children needed vocabulary to be able to communicate in other, including novel environments. The children still needed personal communication systems to enable autonomous communication at any time to learn "to say what I want to say, to whoever I want to say it to, whenever I want to say it, however I choose to say it."

So, we began to use the aided language stimulation techniques suggested by Goossens, Crain, and Elder in their book with both activity-specific displays and the children's personal communication books and dynamic display devices. As we attempted to converse using these communication books and devices throughout the day, we realized how annoying and difficult the vocabulary organization was to use. Parents, colleagues, preschool staff, and other communication partners provided copious critiques, questions, and suggestions as they struggled to model genuine messages. Many modifications to the language organization were tried over the next few years, some abandoned, some kept, but we were always looking for ways to more efficiently meet varied communication requirements. I always thought, "I'm reviewing the situation . . . I think I'd better think it out again."

My biggest challenge came when we began to share our work with aided language stimulation using multi-level, dynamic display communication books (pre-PODD complexity) with other professionals during the mid to late 1990s. I specifically remember a devastating dinner at our national AAC conference.

We were excited by our observations of children with complex, multiple disabilities self-initiating communication for a variety of purposes with their families and friends in a way we had not previously seen. We naively thought others would be interested in discussing our interventions that had brought about this progress. We expected professional feedback, questions, and even criticism of our work, but not ridicule.

Our workshop presentation was filled-to-capacity, and we had thought-provoking questions and discussions in that forum, but then came the night of the conference dinner. My co-presenters could not attend this social event, and, fortunately, I was sitting with other friends from the AAC community. One of the usually fun features of this event was a talent competition. It turned into a nightmare for me as one of the groups decided to perform a song including lyrics specifically making fun of our multi-level books, singing, "Turn the page, turn the page, turn the page, turn the page, turn the page, turn the page, turn the page. MORE." This group of people were known to be passionate advocates of a specific AAC system that emphasized minimizing the number of selections to generate each word. The fact that what they said was incorrect, that I could professionally point out that even these early multi-level books did not link together that many page-turns or require so many selections to access a word like

MORE, did not matter at that time. What I felt in that moment was the eyes of the room move toward me, adrenaline pumping, the fight-or-flight response stimulated, panic rising in my head and chest! Then I felt the hand of a highly respected colleague, a friend, moving onto my knee under the table, reassuring me, comforting me, giving me strength. "Don't react to them." For the next few minutes (which felt a lot longer) of devastating attention, I used self-talk to keep it together, "Keep your face blank," and "Do not cry," I told myself.

After a moment like this, it can be tempting to go back to your safe space and never try to share your work again. Or, returning to a safe space, surrounded by people who share your understanding, can be helpful to re-energize you and restore your confidence to go back into the wild. I get my inspiration and energy from two main sources:

1. Spending time with the children and families and hearing the stories or seeing children communicating something unexpected, expressing their personality and the joy of interaction.

2. Discussing possibilities and problem-solving with people who share a similar understanding and passion.

Critique, feedback, and questioning have been essential to the development of the PODD communication system. I could not have refined and learned without evaluation and reflection from professionals, family members, colleagues, and other community members over the decades of development before the PODD resources were published. Fortunately, most feedback was presented constructively, but it can still be challenging to receive negative feedback on something you have invested substantial time and effort developing. It has taken me many years to learn how to deal with negative comments and how to analyse feedback to refine the effectiveness of the intervention, the design of the PODD resources, and/or the content or delivery style of information in PODD trainings.

The first commercially available PODD resource was published in Australia in 2007 with the support of the Cerebral Palsy Education Centre and a financial grant from Telstra Australia. The publication of PODD resources enabled more people to adopt the system without the hundreds of hours, knowledge, and the expertise required to develop the individualized PODD book or page set from scratch.

My life has been playing catch-up ever since. I receive requests to translate PODD resources into other languages and paper sizes and to make the electronic PODD page sets available for multiple kinds of software and apps. The work continues as I develop, teach, and mentor PODD trainers to offer PODD workshops around the globe. My passion and energy as a clinical speech pathologist and an AAC educator still come from the children, families, and adults who use AAC. Fortunately, I have been able to license other people and organizations to publish and distribute the PODD resources, allowing me to focus on the resource development and training for PODD as a product.

Recommendations

If working primarily with children learning to use AAC, find opportunities to meet and interact with adults who are more competent users of AAC. While it is important to know the general destination of your work, be open to how you might get there.

Be open to feedback and learn how to separate the important content from the style of any negative criticism. These questions may help you.

1. Do they have a valid point?

    a. If yes, is there something you could do, a strategy you could integrate into your system? Be prepared to review the situation and think it out again.

    b. If no, and you can say, "I already tried or thought of that," then ask how you can explain or demonstrate the difference.

2. Do you have a shared understanding of what you are trying to achieve, the purpose of AAC?

    a. To quote U.S. State Department spokesman, Robert McCloskey, "I know you think you understand what you thought I said but I'm not sure you realize that what you heard is not what I meant."[9]

    b. If no, how can I develop this shared understanding? What education, training, or experiences may help?

My wish for you is that you have shared experiences that inspire your passion for AAC.

---

[9] Attributed to Robert McCloskey, U.S. State Department spokesman, by Marvin Kalb, CBS reporter, in TV Guide, 31 March 1984, citing an unspecified press briefing during the Vietnam

Ways to Connect with Me

Website: http://podd.com.au/

Gayle Porter is a speech pathologist with 40 years of experience working with people who have complex communication needs. Gayle is internationally known for her work developing the Pragmatic Organisation Dynamic Displays (PODD) communication books and page sets for electronic speech generating devices. In 1996 Gayle received the Speech Pathology Australia, Elinor Wray Award in recognition of outstanding clinical contribution to the profession of speech pathology, and in 2007 she was the first recipient of the Australian Group on Severe Communication Impairment (AGOSCI) award for services to Australian AAC.

You Tell Me

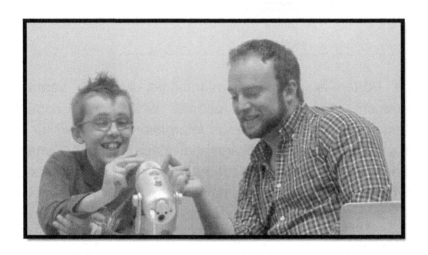

Lucas Steuber, MA Applied Linguistics, MS, CCC-SLP

"Life can only be understood backwards; but it must be lived forwards."[10] ~ Søren Kierkegaard

* * *

It's 11 p.m. on Saturday, January 2021, and I'm staring at a blank page. Anyone who knows me will agree that's unusual. Words are not something that typically come slowly to me; in ~~fact, I've landed myself in~~ trouble more often than I'd like to

[10] "Soren Kierkegaard Quotes." BrainyQuote.com. BrainyMedia Inc, 2021. 21 March 2021.
https://www.brainyquote.com/quotes/soren_kierkegaard_105030

admit by letting my words outpace my thoughts. I'd like to say that I'm preoccupied, or I can't think of any interesting stories to share, but in reality, I know the truth: it's because, for this book, I've been asked to write about myself in the context of my career, and my career isn't about me. It's about the people I serve, their lived experiences, and those moments of joy at every minor stage of growth. It's about the beautiful infinite generability of language, the right people have to it, and everything it can unlock. It's about seeing a need—a gap in training and technology and understanding that's marginalizing what is arguably the world's most underserved minority group—and knowing that in some small way I can grab the world and push it closer to justice. I don't think about me. I rarely even match my socks.

But that's a cop out, and the reality is we *do* need to tell our stories as professionals. I have the best job in the world, and this industry—this clinical space—is in desperate need of more people willing to put their souls into it. There was a time when I didn't even know this field existed, and a time after, when I needed to be convinced it was the right fit for me. Now, if you'll allow, let me convince you. I'll take a moment to stop living facing forward and, like Theseus (son of King Aegeus of Athens) tracing back his ball of yarn through the labyrinth of Crete, I'll take the return journey and see if I can uncover some clues. In the end, only you can tell me if I've found them.

Let's start where all stories do: at the beginning

When I was growing up, my family always expected me to go into business. Expect is actually a generous term; an MBA was practically a prerequisite for membership (although a JD or MD would be reluctantly accepted). I wasn't really into business though—an irony that is not lost on me given that, for years now, I've been working in industry, which is the colloquial term for clinician who now makes stuff to sell. My rebellion played out in short, tentative baby steps. I liked computers, and my family thought computers were the business of the future; it was the perfect cover. On top of that, I was playing a deeper game; what I really liked was math. There is something so elegantly beautiful about pure fact, about an equation or a theorem that lines up just perfectly and resolves itself like a game of Tetris. Order and structure from chaos–the very definition of the universe wrought whole by logic alone.

So, there I was, in February of 2003, at the University of Oregon happily studying my math and smiling my way through the coding courses (or completely butchering my way through, as I discovered when I started to work with *real* programmers)—and suddenly, *outrageously*, I was told that I needed to take courses in an "unrelated topic area" to fulfill some requirement for *whatever, who cares.* The nerve of those people. I'd done all this work out-maneuvering my family—you know, those people paying my tuition—and here I was scuttled regardless. Anyway, I decided to knock a few out in a term, found the few that fit my schedule, and enrolled in a course in Etymology(the history and evolution of language)and Syntax. Syntax I recognized from computer science terminology and the Etymology course, if I recall correctly, I chose because it was timed so that I could sleep in.

Listen, I'm not sure what a spiritual experience is—again, as mentioned above, I'm not a particularly introspective guy. My working hypothesis, however, is that I pretty much had one. Language was—is—*beautiful.* It's math played by a symphony, every note you hear structured and rule-bound, yet unique. Sentences can be short. Snappy. You can catch someone's attention, draw them in. Then, when you're ready, you can unleash a long sentence—structured, engaging, informative—and feel truly heard, truly understood. Math is a means by which we can understand the universe, but language is a means by which the universe expresses itself.

I was hooked.

Five years later my course was well and thoroughly set. As of March 2009, my family still (mostly) talked to me, I'd finished my BA in Applied Linguistics, and found my niche in a master's program. I had found the union of my two loves in the form of Corpus and Computational Linguistics and was writing my thesis on disordered language structures among individuals diagnosed with Schizophrenia using a massive database of transcripts. I had great relationships with the faculty, a fantastic thesis advisor—which I'm able to say in retrospect, my sentiments were slightly different immediately after my defense—and I was doing what I loved. I met my now wife, also in the master's program, and made all kinds of friends among exactly the kind of wacky and bizarre people who get master's degrees in linguistics.

When assembling my thesis committee, university rules required that in addition to my advisor I choose one member of faculty from within the Linguistics department and one member of faculty from a different field. I asked around, wondering who I should ask to join, and I was told I should get a speech-language pathologist.

"A what?"

From the Communication Sciences and Disorders program.

"The what?"

I made it through a bachelor's and almost all the way through a master's degree in linguistics without knowing speech-language pathology existed. My immediate assumption was that communication science had something to do with journalism or giving speeches or something. I made an appointment with the recommended faculty member, an expert in neurogenic language disorders, and showed him a draft of my findings. He told me it reminded him a bit of Broca's Aphasia, partial loss of the ability to produce spoken, manual, or written language.

"Who's what?"

I started to do some research and—well, here we go again.

You might know the feeling of a hard Individualized Educational Plan (IEP) meeting. On this day, in April 2014, I had just come out of a *hard* IEP meeting; lawyers on both sides, a mediator in between, a large interdisciplinary team, and … me. Me, in my second year working in what was an absolutely fantastic school district in Oregon. I'd been sure that I was going to be working in the hospitals until a fateful practicum assignment in graduate school where I met a clinician who remains my mentor to this day. I worked with Sonja, a young girl with Rett syndrome, for whom I built my first homemade eye gaze system to replace the hulking beast that insurance wouldn't replace. I worked with Jeff, selectively mute and unwilling to come to school for three years until I mailed him a letter from Hogwarts inviting him to join (we're still in touch). I wrote Joe Biden on behalf of a student with a disfluency and he actually wrote back with encouragement. I made a ton of mistakes, but I learned a lot and I did my best, and most of the time, my best worked.

But I was frustrated by the bureaucracy, by never feeling that I had enough time, by the caseload—which I came to learn was actually relatively *low* at this district. I later met an AAC specialist who was on the IEPs of 182 different students. More than anything, though, I was frustrated by something systemic; I worried then, and I worry now, that we're creating an alternative system when we should be creating a system of alternatives. I mean that in two senses: both the structure and logistics of special education (and education generally), but also in terms of the AAC systems we design and implement. If gradual conformance to typical social and developmental standards is the ostensible goal of individualized education, then we are already hobbled by the fact that we are attempting to achieve that while offering radically different tools and experiences to the students we seek to serve. If a square peg doesn't fit in a round hole, who's fault is that? The peg, the hole, or the person trying to jam it in?

I worked with many students and had rewarding experiences; including one with a student whose parents were in the room.

Becoming an Exceptional AAC Leader

I'll never forget when his mother turned to me, looked me in the eye, and said:

"You told me this system would bring some light into my child's life, but all you people do is help him come to grips with the dark."

I sat in the parking lot for a long time after that—long enough that it was now morning in India, where the app he was using was designed. I did some smartphone sleuthing and found a phone number with at least four more digits than I was used to seeing, dialed, and just let loose. I talked about language systems. I talked about access. I talked about symbols, and colors, and funding, and even the placement of little bits in their menu options that I didn't think were right. The person on the other end of the line, who is now a close friend, patiently took notes. Eventually I hung up. Ten minutes later the CEO called me, told me nobody's ever done that before, and offered me a job.

A year later, I'd helped boost the strengths and whittle down the weaknesses of their namesake application (Avaz) and had launched another one, a collaboration from scratch called FreeSpeech. It was the perfect opportunity—all that work with computers, math, and language coming together into a beautiful whole with an amazing team. We were the first application for special education to ever be featured in the #1 slot by Apple in the iOS App Store and won the CES Best of Show award in the category of Technology for a Better World.

Meanwhile, I felt like four children in a trench coat trying to buy tickets to an R- rated movie. An imposter. There was no way that we'd done that, right? I hadn't helped with that, couldn't be me.

That feeling doesn't go away, but you learn to harness it. If you don't feel adequate, then go prove yourself. If you don't think you know about something, go learn it. I guarantee, if everyone reading this, set aside six months or so of their evenings, they could read every single piece of literature ever published on AAC. It's a young field with an impossible mandate: to tackle defining and facilitating the infinite, beautiful fractal that is human language, which is poorly understood even among neurotypical learners. Meanwhile, we get to work through all of the developmental and cultural complexities of vocabulary choice, developmental literacy, and pragmatics. All of this is, of course, done on bleeding-edge technology that accommodates access methods largely unknown to the consumer public, like eye tracking and brain-computer interfaces. Oh, and I almost forgot—you also get to make sure it works across the entire continuum of human development, aging, motor, and cognitive ability, often in multiple languages, while lives are literally at stake. Easy.

I may still feel like an imposter, but I'm not sure anyone wouldn't with that set of expectations. My motto now: "One impossible problem at a time."

My professional goal as both a clinician and a developer has always been to have the largest possible "footprint" in terms of positively impacting the AAC community. By May 2019, I'd had at least a hand in many of the most disruptive and innovative developments of the past several years: the spread of Avaz throughout India, China, and the developing world; the increasing popularity of voice banking and custom-made synthesized voices; the launch of the first AAC-specific telepractice platform; the localization of Snap Core First, a symbol supported software application, into 13 different languages and waging internal warfare—with a fantastic boss as my ally—to drop the price by 75%, and lots of new hardware development across touch, switch, and eye-tracking access methods.

Meanwhile, I'd founded and grown a private practice, LanguageCraft, (the kids told me what to name it)across three locations with seven SLPs and a board certified behavior analyst (BCBA), and then sold it because I couldn't handle being back in the world of paperwork. I started a website promoting evidence-based practice called SpeechScience, along with a podcast called Talking With Tech that had (still has) thousands of weekly listeners—and then sold that, too. I launched a male recruitment program for the American Speech-Language Hearing Association (only 3% of SLPs are men), and I joined a couple nonprofit boards, including one where I sat next to Temple Grandin, a scientist and author known for her work in autism and animal behavior.

I built and sold AAC hardware and software for a man in Slovenia who kept them in a shed with his goats. I sold eye-tracking devices in cash to Qatar, United Arab Emirates, and Saudi Arabia, and spoke at the first-ever assistive technology conference in Pakistan. I had a running email thread with Noam Chomsky arguing about syntax. I became the kind of person who turns down media inquiries because I can't be bothered and complains when I don't get an automatic upgrade because of my frequent flyer miles.

Of course, I was *also* the guy who had fallen into an open manhole in Nairobi because I wasn't paying attention, who put his car into *airplane mode* while driving to a home health appointment in private practice (translation: the car flew, briefly, then drove no more), flipped the switch to terminate access to the Compass AAC app and infuriated thousands who were already using it, and helped to facilitate Tobii Dynavox's acquisition of Smartbox and then watched it fall into regulatory shambles. Like I said at the beginning—I don't even match my socks.

The point is, I had reached that footprint. I was the director of product at the largest company in the industry, selling into 57 countries with eight very talented people answering to me— and many others answering to them. I worked with incredible software development and clinical content teams with really big hearts. And on December 5th, I walked away. I felt like I could look back in that moment and visualize my life as a canyon—all of my actions and experiences carving it deeper and deeper—and faintly in the distance I could see the high-water mark, like the watershed had broken and I would never get back. I wasn't going to get anything more accomplished without making a change.

11

https://www.oxfordreference.com/view/10.1093/acref/9780198609810.001.0001/acref-9780198609810-e-7700

It was time to tack widdershins[11] again.

I'm sailing against the wind, taking the hard road again. My journey has been carved by this intimately familiar resistance born from 16th century archaic Scottish roots. Such rebellion has been foundational to my ability to innovate. I'm changing course again.

It's three o'clock on a Sunday in June 2021, and the page is no longer blank. I feel like I'm shining; perhaps that high-water mark wasn't there after all. We've just announced the Cognixion ONE—a wearable brain-computer interface paired with augmented reality, definitely the world's most advanced speech generating device—which has been my secret project with some very talented people for the past year. As I type these words, a neural network is training the predictive language model in another tab; that takes time, but I still have plenty. Let's face forward again.

I'll let you in on a secret: at the very beginning, I lied. It's always been about me too. I love this work. Yes, I am passionate about serving the population, and building better tools, and banging away at the walls of the cognitive and bureaucratic jail we've placed ourselves in as related health professionals. I do all of that for the greater good—but also because it's better than coffee for getting me out of bed in the morning. Every day is a new adventure—a new development, a new skill mastered, a new person met, a new life changed. By my best calculation, only about 11% of the people in the United States who could benefit from AAC are even aware that it exists. Who could pass up an opportunity to explore language and technologywhile serving the common good, especially in light of the incredible opportunity for growth that lies ahead?

I'm often surprised when I see or hear negative attitudes in our field. Don't people understand what we're up against? All the reasons I love this field are the same reasons why awareness is so low and device abandonment is so high. It's complicated, it's ill-understood, it's paperwork-intensive and costly. More than anything, it's intimidating—due at least in part to the rancor between professionals defending their different brands or language-system tribes, which becomes almost comical to watch when you get deep enough in to realize that yes, some people are approaching AAC *wrong*, but it's abundantly clear that nobody is approaching AAC perfectly *right*.

The truth is that the only competition in this field is awareness. People think we're fighting for a *slice of the pie* when the reality is, I'm not baking a pie to sell to you, I'm building a kitchen. Bake your own pie, or come build with me; believe me, there's no poverty of people in need. We're just trying to reach them and be sure they understand that *we know they are whole,* we're not trying to *fix* them; we're offering a tool to more safely and capably interact with their lived environment—no different from shoes, or glasses, or a warm winter coat. Then, more than anything else, we need to listen.

The other day I had a video call with a friend with cerebral palsy. He's using an eye-gaze system I helped build, with software made by a team I managed. Beyond enjoying his friendship, I also like to check in and see what feedback he might have. Now he's considering our new wearable. When the call started, we said our respective greetings and then he said, "What do you want to talk about?" I was honored to be able to say the three words that define who I want to be as an SLP, as an AAC specialist, and as a human:

"You tell me."

My Community

Watch my interview with Mai Ling Chan on Cognixion's What's New? What's Next? in AAC:

Ways to Connect with Me

luke@lukesteuber.com

www.lukesteuber.com

Lucas Steuber is an applied linguist and speech-language pathologist who now works in development of AAC and assistive technology. He began his career working in the schools before moving into private practice, where he specialized in low-incidence disorders. Since then, he has served as the clinical director and/or director of product at several major AAC industry organizations, including Avaz, Tobii Dynavox, Cognixion, and others. He has twice won the CES Technology for a Better World award for his AAC and AT designs and also serves in a strategic planning capacity for the Autism Society of America.

Taking Time to Listen

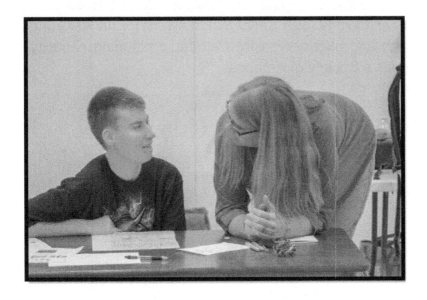

Jane Odom, MEd

Photo by Chase Odom

* * *

My dream was to be an artist, but that idea did not go over too well with my parents. My mom was convinced that only *weirdos* went to art school and my employment opportunities would be limited. As a compromise, my parents allowed me to apply to the Tyler School of Art in Philadelphia, Pennsylvania. This is Temple University's art school. I did not get in but was offered admission to Temple with the ability to transfer to the Tyler campus after my freshman year.

As I started to explore classes, I thought becoming a teacher might be something I would enjoy doing. I majored in education. The program allowed me to get a dual degree in both elementary and special education.

All was going great. I loved my classes, joined a sorority, and became active on campus. Going to school in Philadelphia was great fun with lots of wonderful culture, museums, festivals, and more.

Then came time to do my student teaching. My first placement was in a school that served students with cerebral palsy and other physical disabilities. The class I was in had about ten students who had a variety of physical challenges. I had never worked with kids with special needs before and had no idea what I was doing.

Unfortunately, the lead teacher had the expectation that I knew what I was doing, and instead of giving me guidance, spent most of the time criticizing me. It was so discouraging. She tried to fail me and suggested that I NEVER teach....EVER. I sat down with my professor and she agreed I had completed all my required hours and objectives and ended giving me a B in the class. But those words stung. I questioned my aspirations and myself.

My second placement was amazing. I was placed in an inner - city school with an experienced teacher who was so encouraging and patient. She taught me so much and gave me back some of the confidence I lost in the previous placement.

I graduated with a dual degree in Elementary and Special Education from Temple University in 1987. I was excited to get into the classroom and work with children. I began teaching in inner city Philadelphia. It was a tough job, there was not a lot of funding, and I was often picking up extra shifts as a waitress to make ends meet. This allowed me to get what I needed for my classroom. I remember the ditto fluid to run copies was like gold, and there never seemed to be enough paper, books, or other needed materials. However, I loved the students and tried to create a fun, learning environment with what I had available.

One day, my college academic counselor called about a new program at the university. Funding was available for a small set of students to work at a graduate level in the field of augmentative and alternative communication (AAC). I had no idea what that was, but was willing to explore, especially since I would be fully funded.

Even though I had limited knowledge of the use of AAC, the beginning classes helped us explore a variety of tools that were available to help students. I was intrigued, because at the time, there was not a lot of technology available. Students who were nonverbal often had lap trays on their wheelchairs with a variety of keyboards and /or pictures that they would point to or look at to communicate.

One of the classes in the university program was called ACES (Augmentative Communication Empowerment and Support). It was a two-week seminar where students, professionals, and adults with communication disabilities came to campus and stayed for two weeks in the dorms while attending classes on a variety of topics.

I came in on the first day of training wide-eyed and ready to learn. Little did I know how this day would change the direction of my career. Bruce Baker, world-renowned creator of the Minspeak® system, was there to train us on the language system he had developed called Semantic Compaction. It was a way to code language so those using it could reach any word in three hits or less. I was able to borrow an AAC device called a Liberator. I spent the next day at my apartment complex's pool learning the language patterns and icon meanings. I loved it.

During those two weeks, I got to know a variety of amazing people including actual AAC device users. I learned how capable and unique each person is and about a variety of access methods, device settings, and why core vocabulary is so very powerful.

Each word had a unique icon sequence. Icons on the system were chosen because they could represent a variety of categories and vocabulary. For fun, I created a game and gave everyone involved in the program their own icon sequence.

The staff member in charge loved the game and, ultimately, I was encouraged to keep going, encouraged to consider this field as my career path. Little did I know my professors noticed: Dr. Diane Bryen and Dr. Amy Goldman were integral in helping me discover this amazing field of study.

I was asked to come back each summer as the communications instructor. Each ACES session was so different depending on who attended. Although I was there as an instructor, I learned more from the attendees than they could have possibly learned from me.

The first year, I was paired with one of the students who used AAC. This young man, in his 20s, had cerebral palsy and used a wooden board with the alphabet on it to communicate. He would point to letters to spell his message. He was very quick and got irritated with me because he was usually on word four when I was still figuring out the first word he spelled.

At this time, his staff was trying to convince him that he should live in a nursing home due to his disability. As I eventually learned, this man was incredibly intelligent and had no desire to live in a geriatric nursing home for the rest of his life. But, since his communication method required a knowledgeable communication partner who took the time to spell out his message, his attempts often went unanswered.

In the early 1990s, he came to ACES. We got him a communication device, and my job was to help teach him the language on the device. We practiced and practiced, and he caught on quickly. He began telling his staff exactly what he thought of their idea of living in a nursing home. His voice was heard.

In 1993, President Clinton appointed this young man, Bob Williams, as the commissioner for the Administration on Developmental Disabilities (ADD). He presided over a network of services designed to increase the independence, productivity, and community inclusion of Americans with disabilities and their families. Even with all these responsibilities, Bob sometimes returned to ACES for graduation, sharing his story and inspiring others. Could he have done this living in a nursing home? I think not.

This had—and still has—such a powerful impact on me. I learned how important it was to have a voice and learn to use it. I could see firsthand, how an AAC device could change someone's livelihood. I wanted to help more people do this.

However, at the time, my reach was limited. I had moved from Pennsylvania to South Carolina. Funding was not available from the state Medicaid program for devices and schools claimed to have limited resources. Many students who could have benefited from the technology were not given the opportunity to get the technology.

I began teaching at a high school. I had one student, Francis, who was 18 years old. Francis had cerebral palsy, which limited his vocalizations. He was smart, creative, and had a great sense of humor. Because he had no way to communicate effectively, very few got to know him. Francis would make a certain face when he was upset. Classroom staff called it his pineapple face. One day, Francis and I were working in the library and he made that face. We played the "yes"/"no" game where I asked a variety of questions to determine what was wrong. He looked up for yes and down for no. After multiple questions, I figured out that something was very wrong, and he wanted me to call home. I called home and Francis' dad answered. I explained what had happened in the library, and his father didn't know what could possibly be upsetting his son. I looked over at Francis to see him absolutely cracking up. It was all his way of playing a practical joke on me. He really needed a way to express himself.

I started the process of writing an AAC evaluation with his speech-language pathologist (SLP) to submit to his insurance company. I also began doing AAC evaluations for other local school districts. These experiences led to presenting at the state's Assistive Technology Conference. After my presentation, an entrepreneur named Chip Clarke, who had a business called Assistive Technology Works (ATW), approached me. He asked if I would consider leaving my teaching career to work for him as a consultant? I jumped at the opportunity, and my fulltime AAC career began.

ATW was a reseller of a variety of products including AAC devices, environmental controls, classroom supports, and even one of the first eye-gaze systems. Chip was a businessperson, and he taught me about the business side of the industry. This job laid the groundwork for the rest of my career - and I loved it!

As you can imagine, with technology, the hardware is constantly changing. When I first started in this area, AAC devices had static displays with paper overlays. Many people still had paper overlays taped onto wheelchair trays and symbols were reorganized constantly. The first actual devices I worked with were large, boxy, and voice choices were limited. Perfect Paul and Kit the Kid were standard built-in synthesized voices.

Then came dynamic displays. Programming was more versatile and could be easily customized. Funding became a bit easier, but still not 100% recognized by insurance companies or state funding sources. Voice choices were improving.

South Carolina at that time was not funding any type of assistive technology. Parents who knew their rights were the only ones who managed to get technology for their children and usually had to threaten to sue the local school district. My territory also included North Carolina and Georgia. At least these states recognized AAC as a medical necessity.

While working for ATW, I got a call from Thompson, Georgia to help out a client with ALS that had just gotten his AAC device, the Pathfinder. I met Pastor Willie and his wife, Valerie, at a training that I was doing. I learned that Pastor Willie had his own church and was interested in staying active. I took some extra time and showed him a couple of tricks to help him preach again. We explored the use of notebooks in the device that would allow him to compose his sermon. I taught him how to speak it either all at once or one sentence at a time. We also looked at how to program in pauses in the sermon as he was speaking it from the notebook. Apparently, Pastor Willie's church was quite demonstrative, so adding pauses for parishioners to respond was important. After a couple of weeks, I got a call from Valerie inviting me to hear Pastor Willie preach. No way was I going to miss out on that.

My husband Art and I piled the kids in the car and headed out to church. The congregation welcomed us with open arms. My youngest son, Chase, was about three years old and quite a friendly child. He and his brother, Mason, went to bible study with all the other children and then returned for the service. We sat in the back pew as my husband used a wheelchair and since the church was so small, it was the only place he could fit.

The choir sang and then Pastor Willie began to preach. The joy on his face was contagious and, as he spoke his sermon using his AAC device, he would often say "Amen" or "Praise the Lord"' and the congregation would repeat the phrase. My youngest son could not wait until he could also yell out. He got so many high fives as we left. We went to the family's home afterward and the entire family was so thankful and excited that Pastor Willie could continue despite losing his voice. These moments reinforce the power of having a voice.

But, as life changes, so do our goals. I decided to leave ATW and was fortunate enough to get a couple of job offers in the industry. Because of my time at Temple University and the ACES program, I really respected the Prentke Romich Company (PRC). I was fortunate enough to land a fulltime consulting position with them.

My husband Art and I talked one day about where we would like to go on vacation. I mentioned that I would love to see the Grand Canyon. He said if that territory ever became available, I should take it. Guess what happened? Eventually, the company needed someone with experience in Arizona. I was in the home office in Ohio when I found out and immediately called my husband to ask if he would be willing to give up his job and move across the country, he said, "Yes!" I applied for the transfer, and, in 2004, the company moved my family and me out to the desert.

Arizona has an amazing AAC community, and at that time, it also had great state funding. We were barely settled into our new home when I was invited to a community group called Out and About, created and organized by two speech-language pathologists, Deanna Wagner and Dr. Caroline Musselwhite (read Caroline's story on page 1). This group met after school, out in the community and encouraged AAC device users to learn to speak to people who may never have met anyone using AAC.

Both of these amazing therapists are not only skilled with AAC but are also highly experienced with implementation and how to motivate students. They freely share all their knowledge, and I learned so much from working with them both.

Then the new thing that came on the market was the iPad. It was smaller, sexier, and looked more mainstream. It was also more affordable. Many viewed it as one-size-fits-all. It was assumed that any student could have and use AAC on an iPad. This did not account for durability, access methods, or product support. Although I was working as a consultant, I began exploring educational materials and techniques, true to my teaching background. This was back when a company called IntelliTools was in every special education classroom. I began working with this company on a statewide project where we looked at using IntelliTool software to help students learn to be better communicators and other educational objectives. Suzanne Feit and Caroline Van Howe were in charge of the project. Both were knowledgeable about the software, and also about how students learned best. Again, by teaming up with professionals who I could learn from, I was honing my skills.

PRC asked me to develop some therapy apps to help students learn vocabulary patterns and basic pragmatics. I didn't know a thing about app creation or where to start. When I sat down with my colleague to talk about my fears, he simply smiled and said, "You'll figure it out." And I did. I found a developer and an artist, and created my first app. I ended up creating seven apps for the company, and each got better as I learned what would work best for our students.

It was during this time I became very interested in implementation, specifically what worked best with students and what did professionals working with AAC need to know to make their job easier. I learned the most when working directly with AAC users. In Phoenix, I was able to work directly in classrooms as well as with families at our Out and About groups. These groups are still active today and meet once a month in the community. They have expanded to a group downtown and one on the west side of town. Out and About not only helps students learn to communicate with those in the community who are not familiar with AAC, it helps spread the message of what AAC is and how to be a successful communication partner.

My next professional challenge for PRC was to develop a website to help parents, teachers, and therapists support their students using AAC. The AAC Language Lab was born in 2008.

I teamed up with some incredible colleagues to create this site, and I have been managing the site ever since. It is truly my dream job. The site is constantly changing and growing, as are my professional skills. For instance, I bought a book about HTML and learned new skills including basic coding and video production. It was truly like learning a new language and it took me a while to become efficient, but now, I can do much of my needed coding without having to ask for assistance.

All in all, it has been a journey and through many ups and downs, the website is now on its second edition. It is challenging and exciting to talk to professionals out in the field about what they need and how the website can help them. I love to find fun, engaging activities that get students excited to use AAC.

The AAC Language Lab website has also allowed me to be creative. It allows me to showcase new materials and techniques. I did not start out with any specific plan for my career but as I look back, I can clearly see how implementation has become my focus.

The Lab has also allowed me to mentor both AAC device users as well as up-and-coming AAC professionals. I love working with those just out of school and starting their careers. Many have had little or no exposure to the field of AAC, but with a little encouragement and training, many realize how rewarding this path can be. The more people are willing to learn, the more they can accomplish.

Generally, many who choose to focus their career on AAC do it for the sheer joy of giving someone a voice. The AAC community is also one of inclusion, and information and encouragement are freely shared.

I am thankful every day for a career that allows me such growth and fulfillment, and I'm touched by the support and friendship the AAC community has offered me, particularly in difficult moments of my life.

One such moment was July 3, 2018, when Art, my husband of 18 years, passed away at the age of 46. He had muscular dystrophy which caused his muscles to deteriorate. I can't say his death surprised me, but I just didn't expect it to happen when he was so young. We donated his body to science (as per his request), and he insisted that I not have a big funeral.

To honor him, we created a hashtag #ROK4ART (Random Acts of Kindness for Art), and the response was overwhelming. Colleagues from all over the United States, Canada, Israel, Australia, and Europe did random acts of kindness in Art's memory. For the next month or so, I would open social media and see yet another kind act someone posted. So many people I knew from trainings and conferences reached out to honor my husband.

Going even further, my dear friend, Sheri Predibon, MS, CCC-SLP, offered her home so we could have a simple celebration of life for Art. My AAC family from all over Arizona, as well as family and friends from other parts of the country, came for the potluck party. We laughed, we cried, and watched video tributes people sent. I am so grateful for colleagues I call friends, and for their support through this very difficult time. I can't think of very many industries that come together to support one of their own in the way this industry supported me and my family.

Recommendations

Thinking about the AAC community and its far-reaching impact brings me to a few simple recommendations for those of you interested in following a career path in AAC.

1. **Get involved.** You can join a local, national, or international group of professionals and people using AAC. Talk to people, ask questions, and learn all you can.

2. **Attend conferences.** The best way to learn about new technology and techniques is to attend one of the assistive technology conferences. There are state, national, and international conferences that are both live and online.

3. **Take advantage of social media.** There are a variety of social media groups on different platforms which can help you connect with others to share information.

4. **Know it's okay to cause a little *good* trouble.** Challenge administrators to consider how important it is to provide needed technology to students who don't have a voice. Challenge parents to think outside of the box and allow their children the chance to communicate independently. Challenge students to learn how important their voice is so they can be who they want to be.

When you hit bumps in the road, I hope you find motivation from these quotes I live by, and now share with you.

"Learning can only happen when a child is interested. If he is not interested, it's like throwing marshmallows at his head and calling it eating." - Katrina Gutleben

"The teacher thought I was smarter than I was, so I was."

- Harry Wong

Ways to Connect with Me

AAC Language Lab

www.aaclanguagelab.com/

Email: jane.odom@prec-saltillo.com

LinkedIn: Jane Odom

Facebook: Jane Odom

Jane Odom is the AAC language lab training and implementation specialist for PRC-Saltillo. Jane represents PRC-Saltillo at regional, national, and international conferences, and she works regularly with SLPs, OTs, educators, and family members to address the needs of people with speech, language, and cognitive disabilities. Jane earned her BS and MEd degrees from Temple University and has more than 13 years of teaching experience in special education. She also was the language instructor for the ACES

(Augmentative Communication and Empowerment Seminar) program at Temple University for nine years where she taught AAC device users alongside professionals about how to use and implement AAC devices in everyday life.

Peer Mentoring: My Journey to Be an AAC Leader

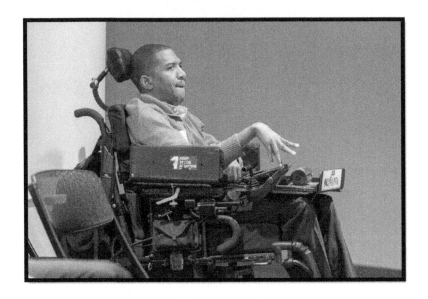

Lateef McLeod, MFA

Photo by Albert Mayson

* * *

I thought my plan was ingenious. I would do my field research as a PhD candidate on the peer mentoring program I helped create some years earlier, with the International Society for Augmentative and Alternative Communication (ISAAC) LEAD committee for young adults who use augmentative alternative communication (AAC).

Peer mentoring, as I have learned in my personal life and through my academic and professional experiences, creates a bridge of understanding between generations of users of AAC and helps people who are new to AAC better navigate real-life circumstances they may eventually encounter.

As a way to help those who use AAC, I became vice president of the ISAAC executive committee and also the ISAAC's LEAD committee chair, positions I held from September 2016 to September 2020, and I had a decisive voice in how this mentoring program operated. At the same time, I was a student at the California Institute of Integral Studies in San Francisco, taking courses and doing all the prerequisite work; my involvement with the peer mentoring program gave me insights I thought I would be able to use to further my academic research later as a PhD candidate, while also expanding the industry's knowledge base.

The ISAAC mentoring program, called Dare to Lead, allowed five people who used AAC to mentor four young adults from around the world who also used AAC. It was an ambitious project, but those of us in the ISAAC LEAD committee were dedicated to pulling it off and establishing a successful and ongoing peer mentoring program within the organization.

We began planning for the Dare to Lead mentoring program in 2016–2017, with the initial idea to create a leadership seminar for the 2018 ISAAC biannual conference in Gold Coast, Australia. We planned it to be a half-day workshop where we, as a committee, offered our knowledge of what we gathered throughout our lives on leadership and advocacy.

Planning for the half-day workshop was mostly straightforward. We had to coordinate with the ISAAC executive board to make sure all the logistics for the workshop were in place. I, being the main liaison between the executive board and the LEAD committee, was instrumental in making sure everything was in place. I was the one who made sure the room was secure for the workshop and food was delivered for the participants.

The Dare to Lead workshop was a great success. The four mentees who attended had a wonderful time learning about leadership and advocacy. Two of our ISAAC LEAD committee members, Beth Moulam and Yoosun Chung, gave excellent presentations on their experience of leadership and advocacy, which were well received. Both women have exemplary careers and contributed greatly to their respective communities. They are good examples of AAC mentors who inspire their mentees toward their self-advocacy goals.

At the end of the workshop, the four mentees were paired with the five mentors who attended the conference. Because the mentors outnumbered the mentees, one of the mentees was paired with two mentors to work with. I gave all the mentors and mentees the instructions that they should work toward the mentees' goals over the next two years.

For the mentor program, the mentors were told to check in with the ISAAC LEAD committee for quarterly meetings; mentees would join them at the half-year intervals. This way, I thought, the LEAD committee would be kept abreast of the mentoring pair groups' progress. I made sure I was in constant contact with the mentors and the mentees.

For the end of the mentoring program, I asked each mentor and mentee pair to shoot a couple of minutes of video explaining how they worked together to accomplish the mentee's goals for the mentoring program. I envisioned that these videos would be shown at the next ISAAC biannual conference. It was a good plan for a mentoring program, and I thought the people in the program would buy into it.

I thought everything was going well—until it came time for the quarterly meetings.

In the first quarterly meeting, I noticed not all the mentors attended the meeting, which was disconcerting. Thinking it was an issue of time, I tried to poll the group for the best time. When that didn't work, I emailed the individuals who did not show up and asked why they were not attending the meetings. Eventually, one mentor and one mentee dropped out stating they either had a lack of time or they had a lack of interest in the program.

At the half-year quarterly meeting, no mentees attended the meeting and did not respond to my follow-up emails. Seeing this situation, LEAD committee members decided to change the requirements and only require the mentors to attend the quarterly meetings.

Even with that, the attendance for mentors at the quarterly meetings kept declining. Eventually, a year into the program, the LEAD committee decided to discontinue all further quarterly mentor programs and simply ask the mentor and mentee pair groups to record the videos explaining what happened during the mentoring program.

Unfortunately, by then most of the participants were disenchanted with the mentoring program, and I didn't receive any videos from any mentoring pair. That is when I knew without a doubt that most of the participants gave up on the Dare to Lead mentoring program.

The failures related to the mismanagement of the Dare to Lead mentoring program were hard to take. I had high plans for the program, but it did not come to fruition. This was a setback, but it was also a learning opportunity.

Although our first attempt to offer an instructional mentoring program to the ISAAC members who use AAC didn't go as planned, we were able to come together as a LEAD committee and formulate another program that would work better within the parameters of ISAAC, such as organizing an instructional webinar series.

In the new program, called the Pathways to Leadership miniseries, we asked people who use AAC and were leaders in our community, to give lectures on how they became successful in a webinar setting. The leaders we selected for this lecture series had the opportunity to explain at length the different strategies they found effective and successful in their personal and professional lives.

I'm happy to say the ISAAC Pathways to Leadership webinars have been successful with the ISAAC membership, and they were well attended. The ISAAC LEAD committee was also able to take the setback of the Dare to Lead mentorship programs and pivot to the success of the Pathways to Leadership webinar series.

Still, I deeply believe that peer mentoring programs can be instrumental in the development of people who use AAC as they come of age.

Most people who use AAC grow up in a community where they are the only one who communicates with an AAC device. Because they do not see these examples in their day-to-day life, having AAC role models for younger people who use AAC to look up to becomes increasingly important. An AAC role model gives a child or young adult who uses AAC a real-life example of how they can live and operate in the world when they become a mature adult and how they can be positive contributors to their communities.

A child or young adult who uses AAC faces many challenges dealing with a severe disability and has a unique way in which they communicate. Seeing other people in their situation who already went through those challenges can be a source of encouragement.

It was in that vein that ISAAC's LEAD committee and I wanted to develop the Dare to Lead mentoring program and the Pathways to Leadership webinar series. We wanted to provide role models, connecting those who use AAC to a new generation of AAC users.

The desire behind my drive to create the mentoring program and the webinar series was the same desire that led me to pivot my PhD field research to observing and evaluating the self-determination program (SDP) at The Bridge School (while I wanted to do my field research on Dare to Lead, it became unfeasible because the project was short lived). All three programs provide a vital role model experience for young people who use AAC.

The SDP is a great innovative mentoring program The Bridge School developed. The Bridge School itself is a remarkable elementary school educating young children with complex communication needs and teaches them how to use AAC devices. After The Bridge School students learn how to use their AAC devices successfully, they learn self-advocacy skills and are mainstreamed in a regular classroom. The SDP mentoring (program) also pairs The Bridge School students with adults who use AAC to teach and model how to use their AAC devices. These adults are also self-advocates. The two mentors in the program are college-educated and are prime examples of what The Bridge School students can achieve if they work hard.

For my field research, I will interview the two mentors and a collection of adult alumni mentee students to discern from firsthand accounts how the mentor program was effective in teaching self-advocacy and leadership. I will also interview the parents of the mentee students and The Bridge School staff to get a more rounded picture of the SDP impact. I want to focus on the voices of the participants of the SDP in my dissertation and have them explain what The Bridge School and the SDP mean to them.

I am currently a PhD candidate in the anthropology and social change department at California Institute of Integral Studies (CIIS) in San Francisco. I attended CIIS from 2016 and was promoted to PhD candidacy in the second half of 2020, just as my term on the ISAAC board ended. It is a very supportive program, both approving of and encouraging me to do my field research. My dissertation chair, my other professors, and my student cohort all believe in me and my work, which I very much appreciate. When I went through my program, I was introduced to many different ideas and texts that expanded my thinking on disability and other subjects. I was introduced to many disability scholars who came before me and laid the foundation for me to do my academic work. In my literature review, I was able to explore this work and see where I could still contribute to the disability canon. Through their work, I understood the many structural and cultural barriers that people with disabilities face in this society. This scholarship informs my approach to my current PhD field research and how I will look at and evaluate The Bridge School's SDP program.

I am so interested in peer mentoring programs for people who use AAC because of my own experiences as a child. When I was growing up, I hardly had any role models who used AAC and few role models who had other disabilities. As a result, I had to imagine what it would be like when I became an adult because I did not have people to serve as reference points as I determined what my adulthood would mean. I did not know how to conduct myself in things like acquiring a job in a job market that is heavily ableist and understanding how employers hire people with significant disabilities. I would have been grateful if older people with disabilities took the time to show me how to disclose a disability to an employer. I would have definitely benefited from older people with disabilities giving me advice in dating and romantic relationships, which has always been a challenge for me because of my disability. These are just a few examples of how a peer mentor who uses AAC can be instrumental for a child or young adult who communicates with AAC. That is why, in my professional career, I was so excited about starting the mentoring project with ISAAC and studying the SDP at The Bridge School for my field research.

As I assisted in the design of a peer mentoring program for people who use AAC and observed another peer mentoring program at The Bridge School, I noted some key things that I want to recount here.

The first thing I observed while I was running the ISAAC Dare to Lead mentoring program with the ISAAC LEAD committee was making sure we had buy-in with our participants. The LEAD committee and I worked hard to develop a good mentoring program that young adults who use AAC from around the world could benefit from. We made a call for participants, and were excited when we got the applicants we wanted to be part of the program. We assumed that all the participants we selected would be willing to go through the whole mentoring program. The downside was that we didn't check in with them to determine if they had the capacity or the bandwidth to stay committed for the duration of the mentoring program. I will take most of the blame for this mistake because I was the main one who designed the program.

Another thing I observed is the challenge of running an international mentoring program without written commitments from the participants. Without anything to make them commit to the mentoring program, we could do nothing when people decided to drop out later down the line.

Lastly, I also observed that the relationship between the mentor and mentee is key for any mentoring program, and that relationship must be positive for any chance of success.

Thank you for reading my story. I hope you enjoyed it. If you want to read more of my writing and contact me, you can visit my website. I would like to hear new stories of people establishing new peer mentoring programs for young people who use AAC. These types of programs are really needed in the AAC community, and I would like to hear how these programs expand across the country and around the world.

Recommendations

If you are inspired to set up your own AAC peer mentoring program, I encourage you to do it. We definitely need more peer mentoring programs for young people who use AAC.

However, if you decide to take on this task, be sure that you have a good, strong relationship with people with disabilities, especially people who use AAC. That is the most crucial part, because I found that the viability of mentoring programs will be based on the strength of the relationships in the mentoring program.

You also need to coordinate with different groups in the community of young people who use AAC who are in the program. This includes the parents, teachers, and specialists like SLPs that are in the AAC user's life and who will help her or him succeed in the mentoring program. You will also have to work together with the mentees' parents, teachers, and speech-language pathologists to make sure the mentee has a good experience in the program.

You should also pay close attention to whom you choose to be mentors for your program. The mentors should be excellent communicators with their AAC devices and contributors in their community. That way, the mentees can admire the mentors in the programs and will be more likely to emulate the mentors' advocacy and leadership skills as they grow up. That is when you know that your mentor program is doing its job.

My Community

Listen to my interview on the Xceptional Leaders Podcast with Mai Ling Chan:

Ways to Connect with Me

Twitter: @Kut2smooth

Instagram: @Teefstyle

Linkedin: https://www.linkedin.com/in/lateef-mcleod-69b58929/

Facebook:

www.facebook.com/lateef.mcleod

www.facebook.com/LateefthePoet

Lateef McLeod is building his career as a writer and scholar. He has earned a bachelor of arts in English from University of California, Berkeley, a master of fine arts in creative writing from Mills College, and is currently pursuing a doctorate with the anthropology and social change department at California Institute for Integral Studies in San Francisco. He published two books of poetry, *A Declaration of a Body of Love* in 2010, and *Whispers of Krip Love, Shouts of Krip Revolution* in 2020, and is currently writing a novel tentatively titled *The Third Eye Is Crying*. He participated in a number of Sins Invalid performances and is now a cohost of the podcast, *Black Disabled Men Talk*, with cohosts Leroy Moore, Keith Jones, and Ottis Smith, www.blackdisabledmentalk.com.

Phoenix: Rising Out of the Ashes

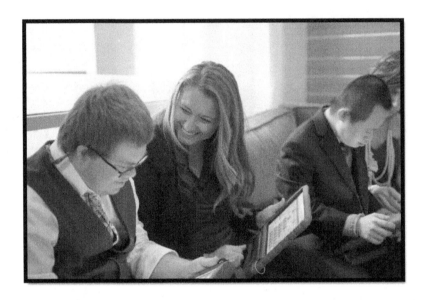

Brandi Wentland, MA, CCC-SLP

Photo by Poise Photography

* * *

I will never forget the phone call I received the morning of Thursday November 8, 2018. My best friend, Jennifer Pearce, called to tell me Paradise, California was on fire. She could see an eerie red blaze hovering over the ridge from her front yard,15 miles away in Chico.

I hurriedly called my mother-in-law. She was panicked. She never panics. Here is a woman who has her own contractor's license, who can cut and haul her own firewood; she is tough, unflappable. She sounded scared, and that scared me.

I grew up in the Bay Area in a big city, east of San Francisco. After high school, I moved north to the small town of Paradise, seeking a place of healing and refuge. Driving into the town, a sign welcomes you, "Paradise, a little piece of heaven here on earth. May it be all the name implies." I later met and married the man whose father built this sign.

After my mom committed suicide in 2006, Paradise became my family, my peace, my sanctuary. This "little piece of heaven" rescued me from my fears, helped me heal, and restored me. It truly was all the name implied.

The town and people of Paradise, and the fire that swept through it, are part of my winding road into speech-language pathology and augmentative and alternative communication (AAC) and my own rise from the proverbial ashes. More specifically, it was a drive in the summer of 2009 up to an annual camping trip to Gold Bluffs Beach that started my AAC journey.

I sat in the backseat of a car chatting with my best friend Jen; our husbands were up front. Jen and I talked about my desire to leave the business sector and return to school to finish my degree. We both knew this was my fork in the road. She was always such a good friend and sounding board. She knew my heart, my passions, and my life story.

At one point she said, "How about speech-language pathology?"

I looked at her with confusion and intrigue. "What is that?"

She responded with excitement, "I don't know. My sister-in-law and neighbor do it. You should talk to them!"

I would later come to know one of those women as my clinical supervisor and the other as a professor. Jen's neighbor became the program director who recommended me for a position to teach AAC at Chico State University beginning in the spring semester of 2021. Talk about a winding road leading to your ultimate fate! Looking back, Jen would say, "I had no idea what I was saying." when she had recommended this path to me.

Within days of returning from our trip, I met two other speech-language pathologists (SLPs), one at a wedding and the other at church. I had never met an SLP in my life. Now, in just one week, I had met two in addition to the two Jen knew. The two women I met had similar responses when I shared my interest, "You should do it! You would be excellent at this! Our field needs you!"

Both women are Christians like me. We prayed together and they continued to pray for me. I am a strong believer. I felt pulled by God to see this through.

After this, two more friends told me they had also always wanted to become SLPs, and they would help me. They prayed for me, too.

How could I not do this? It felt like this was the change I needed and never knew existed. I poured over the local university website, scouring the course summaries and the department page. It was clear. It was time to jump, time to move forward, time to do something my mom would be proud of. If only she were here to do this with me.

Although excited, I was also scared. I was afraid to enroll and attend a university. I had more than 80 units from two junior colleges. The junior colleges weren't scary; they were fun, exciting, and I loved learning. But a big campus, for a girl with undiagnosed dyscalculia, attention deficit disorder (ADD), generalized anxiety disorder, and mild agoraphobia, seemed almost impossible. Just the thought of finding my classes, navigating campus, and parking in a big lot sent me into a tailspin. I was frozen, afraid I couldn't do it and strongly felt "I am not capable."

"I will help you," many friends from my little bubble in Paradise told me, and they truly did! Jen's husband showed me where to park and walked me to my first class. My friend Ashley helped me register for classes and for financial aid, and Jen showed up in the hallways after class to see how I was doing.

In 2012, when I got into graduate school, Jen and Ashley threw me a party I will never forget: a speakeasy with a huge family of friends from Paradise, ready to celebrate with me. These friends, this community, had loved me through hard days, reassured me when I was sure I would flunk out, and consoled me when I simply fell apart from the stress. I never thought I would leave this town. Paradise was home.

So, when my professor, Dr. Shelley Von Berg, someone I admired and respected, suggested I move from Paradise to a big city to get more experience, I hesitated.

"No way!" was my first reaction. My husband had just built our custom home, his dad was a former mayor and on town council, and we led a youth group at our church.

But, this was the same professor who encouraged me to join the American Speech Hearing Association Special Interest Group (SIG) 12, focused on augmentative and alternative communication as a grad student and saw my potential for AAC. While taking her AAC class, I made my own plexiglass E-Tran board to facilitate spelling words to communicate. I loved everything I was learning and even practiced clinical activities on friends.

God kept pulling at my heart, guiding me toward my passion, and in May 2015, after finishing my clinical fellowship with Paradise Unified School District, we moved to Arizona. I would later learn Phoenix was a hotbed for AAC—a place I would meet my mentors and other AAC leaders and trailblazers. Many of them would become colleagues and friends.

Even as life flourished in Arizona, we still had strong ties to Paradise. The 2018 news of a catastrophic fire sweeping through our community devastated us.

We frantically watched the news, monitored social media feeds, and messaged our families and friends as they were experiencing their cars encased in flames and propane tanks exploded around them.

My husband, who was finishing his own degree and had one semester left before graduating, watched in horror as his hometown—the town he and his family built with their own hands—burnt to the ground. While our family and many friends survived, his family home and grandmother's home were gone. A close friend and neighbor could not escape in time and passed away in his home.

Soon after, my husband fell into a deep depression, had complex Post Traumatic Stress Syndrome (PTSD), became suicidal, bonded with his professor and emotionally distanced from me. I found out about the relationship on our 14-year anniversary. I fell apart. How could I survive this without him, without my mom? Why should I? I have no kids, no family and now, no husband. Or so I thought.

My husband and I sought many forms of counseling. We desperately loved each other, but how could either of us survive this? We were both so unhealthy, so broken, deeply depressed, and hurting. He had hurt me beyond anything I could bear. He felt like a failure and that life was no longer worth living.

I cried, I begged God to take me home and end the pain. How could I serve children needing help with this mess I had become? How could I do anything but succumb to the same decision my mom made? I had to end this legacy of pain. Suicide had plagued my family: my great grandfather, grandmother, great aunt and my mom.

Then I remembered the phoenix, the mythical bird that fans flames of fire with its wings and is born again into new cycles of life by rising out of the ashes. My husband always called me his "blue flame," the hottest part of a fire. My intense passion to serve my clients gave me a reason to live another day: they were the wings fanning the flames. My passion for AAC and my colleagues, who saw my potential, increased the heat of the flame. Through this blue flame, this fire, I rose again.

My husband and I also fought to rebuild our relationship. I explained the domino effect of his decisions and detailed what could be lost if our downward spiral continued. This changed his perspective, realizing he hadn't seen the world beyond his own decisions. He returned to counseling and he and I both continue to see the benefit of ongoing professional support.

I took a neurotransmitter test and received medication for anxiety. I learned to breathe. I soon realized I had been walking around holding my breath my entire life, and I could finally exhale. The anxiety meds helped in many ways: I could function without fear of how I would hold it all together, and I could fall asleep without anxiety about tomorrow.

My husband also tested his anxiety levels, and his results were more severe than mine. He opted for herbs instead of medication. The herbal remedies worked well for him. They took a little longer to see the results and were more subtle with slow changes, but they have lasted.

We began to heal individually, and slowly, our marriage healed. We re-discovered each other and created a new relationship. Another life cycle of the phoenix. This healing allowed me to get back on track and continue to pursue my passion for AAC, with my husband's support.

My Inspiration

During my clinical fellowship year, I worked in an elementary school and the same middle school my husband attended as a child.

Even though there was significant need, no child in either school had access to AAC. I spent a great deal of time in a middle school self-contained classroom and volunteered to spend my lunches in that room. This is where I truly unleashed my innate talents and soared like a phoenix. I ignited my internal flame, spread my wings, and felt most connected to my true self.

The teacher, Tami Oliver, shared my passion for getting these kids access to some form of augmentative and alternative communication (AAC). She invited me to attend a three-day Pragmatic Organization Dynamic Display (PODD) course with her. Moved by the course, we decided to do a whole class implementation strategy. I coordinated a plan in which kids in school suspension laminated and cut out PODD books with me. Tami and I trained the paraprofessionals, and they cut out their own books, too.

I was determined to make a change. I wanted every single child in that room evaluated, but my Clinical Fellow (CF) supervisor advised me to take it slow. That year, I succeeded in having four kids evaluated for AAC.

Later in 2015, our first year in Arizona, I began working in Early Intervention (EI). I never thought I could love working with little ones. Teens were my jam. But the collaboration with the therapy team and working in homes with families in daily routines was a dream come true.

This collaborative therapy model matched who I was as a clinician. Once again, though, no child I saw had access to AAC, and no one on my team could tell me how to get them access. I spent my own money to buy a color printer, paper, and ink, and printed out my own PODD books. Families cut the pages and laminated them with me, and as we worked together, I kindled my inner fire.

Eventually, I transitioned to working in-home with teens, adults, and older children. During this time, I met Laurel Buell, an occupational therapist with 35 years of experience in assistive technology (AT), an international presenter with a master's in education, and best friends with Dr. Caroline Musselwhite (read Caroline's story on page 1) and other AAC leaders. Laurel took me under her wing, mentored me, helped me to meet key community leaders, went to conferences with me, and became my AAC co-evaluator. She was there through my first AAC evaluation and is still with me today. She was the first person I told my crazy dream to (starting We Speak AAC, a comprehensive evaluation training resource) and the person who has been there cheering me on and supporting me every step of the way.

Within a year of that meeting, I flew all over the country attending AAC workshops, conferences, and trainings. I met and became friends with some of the trailblazers in AAC. I said "YES!" to every opportunity, including ones that filled me, such as creating my interactive workshop series "Demystifying AAC," and ones I initially shied away from.

The opportunity to mentor Alexis Martinez was one such instance.

While back at my alma mater, California State University, Chico, as the presenter for the annual National Student Speech Language Association (NSSHLA) conference, my professor, colleague, and now friend Dr. Shelley Von Berg invited me to dinner. She encouraged me to work with a young woman she believed had great potential in AAC. In the wake of the Paradise catastrophe and my own fragile state of mind, I felt I would not be able to handle mentoring responsibility and turned down Alexis' application.

Shelly looked me deep in the eyes, "You really should reconsider. This young woman, Alexis Martinez, is all that you are—ten-fold—and you know I don't say that with any disrespect to you."

I valued Shelly's opinion, and trusted the support and confidence she had in me. Her statement gave me pause. "Who is this girl?" I wondered. I asked Shelly to ask Alexis to introduce herself after my presentation. Alexis accepted that invitation.

I was so impressed with Alexis' excitement and the fire I felt within her, I designed an internship for her that I would have wanted at her age—an internship of a lifetime.

Meeting Alexis led to another inflection point. Mentoring her was part of the healing I needed, and she was the one who fueled me when I had no propane left in the tank. She propelled me to do more, be more, and see myself the ways others saw me. It is because of her that We Speak AAC is how most people know it today.

Empaths have the ability to sense the feelings, thoughts, and energies of people, plants, animals, places, or objects. Empaths sense and absorb the energy of those around them, and often experience stress or illness if they are bombarded by too many negative emotions. Empaths can also use their abilities to help others imagine themselves in someone else's situation and connect with them on a deep level.

My gift of empathy and ability to work with families in their homes has shaped me into the clinician I am today. Witnessing the stress, joy, pain, and celebrations families experience, I am better able to support my clients with their family and communication partners, understand their day-to-day struggles, and help them overcome and achieve their goals.

As I have come to discover, my tenacity, drive, grit, and authenticity empowered me to create Demystifying AAC and We Speak AAC and share what I have learned in many other ways.

Recommendations

1. Eagerly and passionately seek out mentors. Don't be afraid to talk to presenters at a conference, email them, and maintain a relationship. Many of the trailblazers and leaders in AAC want to see the next generation carry the torch.

2. Get on a plane. Some of the best AAC conferences and training opportunities will not be in your city, county, or even your state. When the time is right (in terms of health safety), go to Florida for Assistive Technology Industry Association (ATIA), to Pennsylvania for Pittsburgh AAC Language Seminar Series (PALSS), to Minnesota for Closing the Gap, and anywhere you can attend a Language Acquisition through Motor Planning (LAMP) or PODD training. Don't wait for trainings to come to you. You have to be willing to go out and seek what you need.

3. Establish friendships with users of AAC, who are not your clients. Krista Howard and Lydia Dawley (read their stories on pages 130 and 47, respectively) have been close friends since 2017. As a communication partner and friend to two strong, independent, and fierce women who utilize AAC, I have learned so much about how to be a better communication partner, trainer, and clinician.

4. Create a community-based social group for AAC. Dr. Caroline Musselwhite (read Caroline's story on page 1) and Deanna Wagner graciously mentored and guided me in expanding their AAC community-focused Out and About group to the East Valley area of Phoenix, and I have grown immensely as a facilitator of this group. Fostering a community to initiate, establish, and maintain friendships and community involvement for users of AAC will provide you far more than you can ever give.

5. Share what you learn with others. Do not let what you have learned or created stop with you. There are far too many clinicians, parents, users of AAC, teachers, and communication partners who could benefit from what you have learned. Don't wait until you are confident. Sometimes, our best learning comes from when we are teaching. Even when you are at your weakest moment, that next intern, student, or parent could be the person who gives you what you didn't know you needed, when you needed it most.

Much of what I shared with you today required immense vulnerability. It required the willingness to bear some of my hardest moments for the world to see so that others might heal or feel encouraged.

While I have never allowed the world to form calluses over my open heart, I couldn't have overcome some of my fears and shared parts of my story with you without the influence from the extraordinary author Brené Brown. She said:

> Owning our story can be hard but not nearly as difficult as spending our lives running from it. Embracing our vulnerabilities is risky but not nearly as dangerous as giving up on love and belonging and joy—the experiences that make us the most vulnerable. Only when we are brave enough to explore the darkness will we discover the infinite power of our light.[12]

---

[12] Brown, Brené. *The Gifts of Imperfection: Let Go of Who You Think You're Supposed to Be and Embrace Who You Are*, Simon and Schuster

My wish for you is that you realize "what makes you vulnerable makes you beautiful" (Brené Brown), and that you will utilize that vulnerability to connect and share with others.

How does that have anything to do with AAC? I asked myself that same question as I poured this story out onto paper. Your vulnerability is a major part of your journey.

Families have their own journey, as do teachers, therapists, and others with whom you will collaborate. They need to see and connect with your vulnerability for them to feel safe to learn and progress from their area of fear, insecurity, and thoughts of failure.

Embrace your fire, rise from the ashes, help others fan their flame, and discover their wings.

My Community

Listen to my episode on Talking with Tech:

https://www.talkingwithtech.org/episodes/brandi-lee-wentland?rq=brandi

Watch my interview with Mai Ling Chan on Cognixion's What's New? What's Next? in AAC:

(2010). p.20,

Ways to Connect with Me

Website: www.wespeakaac.com

Email: brandi@wespeakaac.com

Facebook: www.facebook.com/wespeakaac

Instagram: @wespeakaac

Podcast: Lotus & Bananas

https://open.spotify.com/show/4rDF4qh1u3DCzCpLi0k37C

Brandi is a speech-language pathologist, adjunct lecturer at California State University, Chico, and U.S. distributor of PicSeePal. Brandi created We Speak AAC, LLC in 2018 to provide mentoring and training for SLPs, school teams, parents, and graduate students. She has a vision to empower more AAC users to become AAC mentors and for providing world-wide access to comprehensive AAC education, training, and coaching through interactive workshops and webinars by leaders in the field of AAC. She is also the cohost of the podcast Lotus & Bananas.

With Brave Wings, She Flies

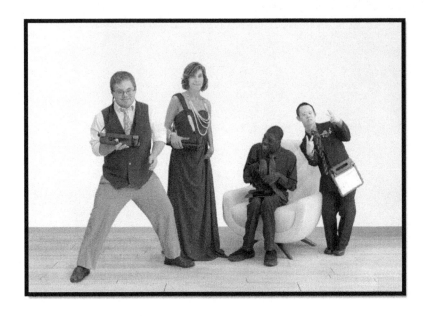

Krista Howard, AA

Photo by Poise Photography

* * *

I like to think of myself as a butterfly. I started off as a caterpillar, crawling inch by inch; but, over time, with hard work, dedication, tenacity, and a whole lot of stubborn determination, I have turned into this beautiful creature with wings.

Sometimes, it surprises people how far I have progressed in my lifetime. It may also surprise them to find out what I've gone through to get where I am. For me, nothing was easy, but rather, many years of life experiences taught me important lessons.

I have cerebral palsy (CP) with learning disabilities, depression, anxiety, and anxiety attacks, but I am still accomplishing my dreams. Having learning disabilities is difficult enough, but throw in cerebral palsy, and it can be quite overwhelming and cause a lot of stress. CP affects each person differently. For me, it affects my left arm and my voice, so an augmentative and alternative communication device (AAC) is my voice. I use this device to do all my talking and making my presentations. I have even had friends ask to use my device to do their own presentations!

I am a single mom, and my son means the world to me. I didn't know I was going to be a mom, but I met a wonderful man, and we got married. We got along well until I became pregnant, then our marriage started to fall apart. Nobody knew how I felt when he left me for another woman, who happened to be my friend. At that time, my mental health diminished, and I was a mess. Despite all of this, I finished college with an associate of arts degree from Estrella Mountain Community College in Arizona, and it was not easy!!

I still remember being in elementary school. I had zero friends because I was so different, and not even my cousin, who was in my class, associated with me—that was probably my most painful rejection. I walked to school alone and stood in line by myself, and I often wondered if anyone would ever like me, or if I would be good enough to have friends. I was depressed, lonely, and desperately wanted someone to talk to. All I had were my classroom aides, and they were there to help with my academic life, not my social life. When I tried to interact with peers, they would walk faster than I was able or ignore me and walk past me. Facebook and cell phones were not a thing at that time.

"Just when the caterpillar thought her life was over, she began to fly."[13] — Barbara Haines Howett

When I was 13 years old, I walked up to my classmate and started talking to him with my device. I was scared to talk to him, but he ended up being special and sweet to me. We talked at lunchtime. I remember smelling the school's food but could hardly eat it. I was looking at him; he was so cute. He had blue eyes, blue like the ocean that my family visited every year since I was born. I felt happy talking to him. We talked about schoolwork, and how much one teacher annoyed both of us. AAC was great to have; it allowed me to talk to him, but I realized I needed more skills to have better friendships. Even though I have better communication skills now, I wanted them back when I was talking to him. I wanted to tell him so many things, but I couldn't spell words like "restaurants" and "movies." I really wanted to share my favorite movie, *The Little Mermaid*, a Disney movie about a mermaid who traded her beautiful voice to become a human for a short time. The Little Mermaid could have used an AAC during that time to communicate instead of using gestures!

---

[13] Howett, Barbara Haines. Ladies of the Borobudur: a Mosaic of Interrelated Stories. Outskirts Press, Inc., 2007.

Using an AAC device can be really challenging, especially if you stop and think about all the words a speaking person says during the day—there are thousands of them. To get a device to say these words, and in sentences, takes a lot of learning, practice, patience, and trial and error. Having done this for more than 20 years, I understand the challenge it is.

Like everyone else, I have many dreams. One of the things I want to do with my life is to support other people learning to use an AAC device for communication. I didn't realize how important AAC was to me until I wanted to communicate with my peers. Since I wasn't really taught literacy and writing skills in school, I was not taught to communicate. AAC would have supported me academically as well as socially. I had been placed in a general education class with special education support, but without individualized instruction in a way that I learned.

In high school, I was placed in a life skills class that focused on cooking and finances—things administrators believed I would need to live independently, but these classes did not prepare me for college. Often, in school, the struggle was that they felt I needed to behave in a specific manner. However, they did not realize that if they had taught me and helped me understand what was going on, I would not have needed lessons in behavior. When I had a writing prompt, I would provide a few words, and my para (educational assistant) would take these few words and complete my assignment for me. I learned how not to work and that others would do the work for me. I did not like it, but it seemed the only way. This did not prepare me for anything but more struggles when I wanted to attend college and get a job. Struggles that continue even today.

At 13 years old, I had the opportunity to go to a summer AAC camp with my only friend, Katie. Katie also had CP, and this was our opportunity to feel somewhat like a normal teenager. We had classes on how to use our devices. Imagine a group of non-verbal youth with machines to talk for them and learning to use them for real conversations! After camp, we went back to our reality of few interactions, loneliness, and a desire to belong. Deanna Wagner MS,CCC-SLP and Caroline Musselwhite, PhD, CCC-SLP (read Caroline's story on page 1), two Arizona-based speech-language pathologists (SLPs) who facilitated learning at AAC camp, saw our need for positive social interactions and created the Fox Girls. It started as a group of three teenage girls getting together to have fun, laugh, and talk. It has now grown into the Out and About group. There are now four Out and About groups in Arizona and many others around the world. I have been volunteering with Out and About for 20 years and continue to help other people learn to utilize AAC for communication.

Working with Out and About helping others learn to communicate is one of my passions. If I can help even one person not feel the loneliness and frustration I have experienced, it is so worth the energy and efforts. I enjoy seeing the ear-to-ear smiles on everyone's faces when one of the people I mentor is able to successfully get their point across.

In addition to Out and About, I also volunteer in schools by providing support to teachers and other staff as they help students learn and use their AAC. I started volunteering when I was 18 and have volunteered in two schools. These experiences have helped me become who I am. I also mentor peers in literacy groups. This gives me practice engaging in social communication with those who share a common interest. You can say that I walk the AAC walk, and I talk the AAC talk!

Making presentations at AAC conferences nationwide has also shaped me. I have done this since I was 16 years old. One time, at a conference in Pennsylvania for the International Society for augmentative and alternative communication (ISAAC), I was asked to give the welcome speech at the president's reception. I was so nervous and afraid that I was going to mess up that I stayed up really late working on it. I kept going over it to make sure it was perfect and also asked my friends to listen to it. When I was in front of everyone, I was shaking so badly I almost peed my pants. Afterward, everyone said that I did an amazing job. This experience was so empowering to me. When it was over, I thought, "That was easy." As I saw how my speech impacted people's lives, I felt even better about helping people. Helping change people's lives is magical!

At another conference, Closing the Gap, I learned I could actually use my AAC to understand literacy concepts. This was surprising because when you look at an AAC device, you only see pictures with words. A verbal person learns to read words and look at the pictures but an AAC user learns to look at pictures, and then learns the words. So, it is backward for us, and we often struggle to identify the words. At this conference, I learned about phonics and how to read words more quickly. I was 32 years old then, and finally was learning to be a better reader. Although I am still faster at communicating by finding the icons, I am getting faster at reading, and I actually understand what I am reading!

Sadly, people judge other people often. We judge the way they look, talk, smell, the clothes they wear, how they hold their bodies, and more. I am often judged as incapable by people because I cannot speak to them. They often treat me like a little child who is incapable of doing anything for herself.

What they don't know, and often don't take the time to learn, is that I want to make a difference in this world. I want to help others who are going through what I have gone through, and I want them to know that they can reach their potential. I am raising a son, with the help of my parents. I have my associate of arts degree and I am currently working on finishing my bachelor's degree. I go shopping. I buy clothes. I buy food. I eat at restaurants. I go to the gym. Mostly, I want people to know that I am as capable of doing things as anybody else. Being nonverbal does not mean being dumb or stupid. I am a person. I hear. I feel. I see. I work.

I get excited when I am out, and people ask me about my AAC device. I love being able to teach others about how I communicate. It is fun to watch their expression when they see how much I can do with something that looks so complicated to them and I make it look easy.

My mentors also inspire me. Dr. Caroline Musselwhite helped me communicate with other people by encouraging me to use my device. She connected me with other individuals who use AAC and prompted me to use my device to make sentences and use core words. She did this by having me participate in motivating and meaningful activities such as Dueling Devices, Out and About, and by talking to me about the importance of using the device.

Tami Taylor MA, CCC-SLP, is another inspirational person to me. She was my speech therapist when I was 14 and came to my house. I was in high school, and it was a big transition time. I was moving out of functional skills classes into an integrated program with academic instruction and resource classes. Tami worked with me once a week for one year. Tami gave me tough love during the sessions. It was hard but I did it.

These individuals did not give up on me when times were hard, instead they pushed me to become the successful young woman I am today. Having people who believed in me is a big part of why I am able to share my story with you today.

I was inspired in other ways, too. When I was in 10th grade, I established a communication circle at my high school to connect and build relationships with my peers and to lessen the loneliness and social isolation I felt throughout my academic career. Our group of five friends met five times a week during lunch and we had fun joking around with each other. During class time, we also learned from each other. This group gave me confidence and happiness. I would not have been able to make it through high school without the support of my communication circle. Perhaps it's not surprising that these high school friends have become my lifelong friends, and I consider them my family.

My goal now is to establish hundreds of communication circles across the nation. I do not want others to experience social isolation. I will do this by bringing my mentoring skills to school districts.

My mission is to be a role model and support system for other users of AAC and their family members. As an AAC mentor, I already provide consultant services to clients, family members, and professionals to support AAC implementation and training. I co-present for webinars and in-person workshops at universities and schools. I helped We Speak AAC start their first student mentorship program. I feel mentoring will change the field of AAC because, after hearing my story, it will help families and professionals work better with users of AAC, while also making them better communication partners.

Before COVID-19, I worked at Gompers, a day program and a school in Phoenix. I worked with members and students with their AAC and trained the staff about AAC. I believe I made a huge difference in people's lives. Since I have a device and used it, that helped others bring and use theirs.

"Butterflies can't see their wings. They can't see how truly beautiful they are, but everyone else can. People are like that too." - Naya Rivera

When I go to AAC-related conferences (I'm lucky to attend and present at many live and virtual events), the people there help me see those wings. They talk with me, compliment me, and share how I have impacted them. I go to conferences to make a difference, to be inspired, and to improve my public speaking skills. Public speaking motivates me to do more because I feel proud and because I want to change lives. When I attend and speak at conferences, I have a larger impact on people who utilize AAC. Conferences also help me with my mental health. People at conferences make me feel I am not different. They talk to me. After I present, I feel excited and motivated.

One such conference was We Speak AAC for Sutter County, California, in 2020. I participated in a live, four-part webinar series where we trained teachers, SLPs, and paraprofessionals about Demystifying AAC. It helped me in several ways. First, I was paid to do what I love while having an impact on others. Second, I was inspired when the county wanted to hire me to work with students and Individualized Education Program teams. After being laid off during the pandemic, it felt great to be asked to do more and to further empower myself. Lastly, it had a powerful impact on my mental health to do something I really enjoyed.

I am also a multimodal communicator, and, because of the work I did as an assistive technology (AT) technician prior to the pandemic, I have LAMP Words For Life, UNITY and TouchChat on various devices, which allows me to communicate with people in different ways.

I like to be busy, but not so busy that I am stressed. When I am busy, it makes me feel like my life has purpose. My friends say I flutter around at conferences, workshops, and in the community like a butterfly. However, butterflies do more than just paint a pretty picture. They pollinate flowers, eat weedy plants, and provide a food source for other animals. My flight path is very similar to these butterflies. I like to make others feel welcome, saying hello to each person in the room, checking in to see how they are doing. Like a butterfly, my presence makes an impact and helps social groups and friendships bloom.

Recommendations

1. Don't give up on yourself or your students/clients. Every human needs at least one person to cheer them on—to shout their name in encouragement during times of progress, stability and also during times of regression. We must believe. And we must keep believing." — Karen Owens, We Speak PODD
2. Establish a peer mentorship program, an Out and About community or another type of community-based social group for individuals using AAC and their communication partners.
3. Establish a communication circle.
4. Model, Model, Model! Provide Aided Language Stimulation (ALgS)
5. Get connected. Join social media groups for support and resources.
6. Build your support network. Your support network can help you follow your dreams and grow with your goals.
7. Follow your dreams.

If you are reading this book, then you have some motivation to follow and accomplish your dreams and goals. You have power in your life. Face your challenges and beat them. Anything is possible when you set your mind to do what you want to do.

My Community

Watch my interview with Mai Ling Chan on Cognixion's What's New? What's Next? in AAC:

Ways to Connect with Me

Website: www.wespeakaac.com

Facebook: www.facebook.com/groups/wespeakaac/

Facebook: www.facebook.com/krista.howard.9

Instagram: @wespeakaac

Email: krista@wespeakaac.com

Krista Howard is an AAC user and is an AAC mentor and consultant with We Speak AAC, LLC. Krista provides support in various virtual social groups including Kate Ahern's AAC Voices and Therapy One's Out and About. Krista has presented at many conferences around the nation sharing her experience as an AAC user and a model for other AAC users. Krista is a mom of a 9-year-old son. In addition to raising her son and working, she is a student at Arizona State University pursuing her bachelor's degree.

While Busy Making Other Plans

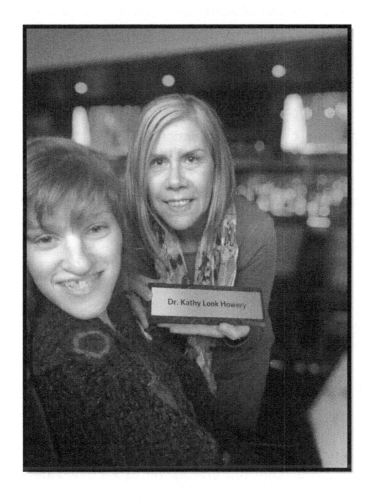

Kathy Howery, PhD

* * *

Can I really do this? And am I mad to even try? Those were the thoughts swimming through my head as I sat at a table in a large room outside the small video conferencing room where I had just experienced my doctoral candidacy examination. I was shaken to the core. The experience I just had in that room was, for lack of a better term, awful. Now I was sitting outside that room awaiting the judgement that was to come down upon me. Would I pass this pivotal test and be able to continue down the path that I had embarked upon, or would I be told I had not measured up, had not answered the round table of questions that I had been faced with in a suitably scholarly and convincing manner? This had never really happened to me before. Certainly, I had been questioned about my understandings and beliefs, but I had never before felt that my answers were not good enough, clear enough, certain enough. On that day, sitting alone outside that large room while my committee deliberated my fate, and indeed in my mind, my worth, I questioned it all—everything.

To understand a bit of how I came to that moment, it is worth going back to the occasions of, shall we say, "serendipity," that brought me to this momentous juncture in my career and, indeed, my life's path. Albert Bandura, the "father" of social psychology[14], and a fellow Canadian, speaks of several instances in his life where his journey veered from what he had been planning due to momentous changes in his life. So too has my life evolved, not always along the path I was seeking but the path that invited me to seek wonderful new opportunities.

---

[14] https://www.stanforddaily.com/2011/03/03/beyond-banduras-bobos/

There were definitely such moments long before engaging in doctoral studies in my late 40s. An early one was when I failed a French exam in my first year of university. That failure led me to leave the arts psychology program and enter into the science psychology program. In that stream I learned about difference, disability, behaviorism, motivation, and many more ideas that were to influence my life in profound ways. Arts had really never been the right place for me; luckily, I failed French and found that out.

Upon finishing my bachelor of science degree, I was not ready to leave the safe and secure world of the university. On to a master's program I would go, but which one? I was encouraged by many psychology professors to stay the course and continue in the path of learning and motivational theory I was on; however, ah here comes the moment, to enter into the master's in psychology program, I would have to write the graduate records exam. The thought of that terrified me for some reason. Looking back now, I can't say why, except perhaps I had a huge lack of self-trust. Whatever the reason, I took the path less traveled at the time and entered into a master's program but in psycholinguistics. A program that only counted your grades (mine were stellar) and did not require writing any exams.

Entering into that program was wonderful. I now could follow my heart and begin to look deeply at communication and language. And look at it from a different lens—one that left behaviorism and Skinner behind—shining light instead on the theories of linguists Noam Chomsky and Dell Hymes. I loved it, and I thrived.

And I found work, work that I loved, with this degree nearly, but not yet, in hand. I actually started my first job as "communication therapist" before my thesis was completely written. The study and approach of my master's degree, coupled with the base knowledge from the psychology degree, proved to be just what I needed to reach children who had only recently been considered educable—children who had, in many instances, been housed in the nearby hospital until this special school had been built. I loved the kids, I loved their parents, and I loved my work. I attended conferences where people were talking about this new thing called augmentative and alternative communication (AAC). I learned to program an Adaptive Firmware Card to let these children engage with computers and show themselves able. I was even interviewed on national radio to talk about the promise of technology for kids with disabilities. Life was good.

Now, I will skip past a few other forks in the road and get to the opportunity that really led me to the fateful day of my candidacy exam, and ultimately, my foray into the world of phenomenological inquiry. I was in my third year of my doctoral program, and even with all my coursework completed, I only now had to figure out my research path. I had entered into the doctoral program with a plan to study universal design for learning (UDL), something that held, according to the texts of the day, substantial promise for changing the face, and perhaps the heart, of education. The trouble was that I could not figure out how to define UDL well enough to study it. The scholarly language would be to "operationalize" the concept of UDL. I was struggling.

Then came the next fortuitous event. Life for me was about to take another unexpected turn. My plans to dig deeply into the promise of UDL in practice became sidelined by what I see now was an ever-more insistent call to go back to the passion of my heart, AAC, and to be compelled to consider what it is really like.

In 2010, I was auditing an educational technology class where I had also been a guest speaker. One evening, Dr. Cathy Adams, who was unknown to me at the time, was coming to talk about her work (Soon after, Dr. Adams became my early muse and my continual mentor on the latter part of my journey).

In that lecture, Dr. Adams spoke to us about the philosophy of technology. She introduced us to Heidegger's (1962) hammer and the McLuhans' (1988) tetrad. The very idea that there was a *philosophy of technology* was beyond anything that I had ever conceived. I was wrapped in something that I can call skeptical fascination. In the class, we were asked to use McLuhan's tetrad to explore a technology that was of particular interest to us. Despite the fact that my paper focused on looking at text-to-speech supports for struggling readers, the technology that I chose was a speech generating device (SGD).

When I was called upon to share my attempt at exploring McLuhan's mode of analysis, I talked of an SGD as *extending* voice, *reversing into* a toy, *obsolescing* communication boards, but I could not imagine anything that it might *retrieve from obsolescence*. In retrospect, it was a very shallow analysis, but the process was so far from the ways I had been taught to consider any technology that I felt like I was swimming in very deep but strangely inviting waters. Happily, Dr. Adams seemed pleased by my attempt, but she was intrigued by the technology that I had chosen. The following week, I found myself having coffee with her. In that coffee shop we continued the dialogue we began that evening in class for some two hours. At the end, she convinced me to take Max van Manen's final graduate seminar in phenomenological writing and research, and my topic of inquiry was to be the experience of using a speech generating device.

Now, let's return to where I was sitting waiting for the verdict from my doctoral committee. Suffice it to say, I passed my candidacy exam that day, but I would say just barely. My choice of inquiry was, to say the least, unusual for someone doing a doctorate in special education, and my committee was skeptical. I, still trying to grapple with this new and unique approach, was likely partially to blame for their skepticism. I was still digging in the dunes myself, trying to unearth what phenomenological inquiry really was, but I was convinced that it was what I wanted, no, what I needed to do, so as the saying goes, I persisted.

That persistence paid off in ways I could have never imagined. I learned so much! I learned that while I knew a great deal about AAC, I really did not understand what it was really like to speak with or through a machine. My work was well received and valued. At the 2016 ISAAC Conference, in a room of hundreds of people, an internationally recognized speaker who had just come from my talk, exclaimed she had just heard the best talk ever about AAC by Kathy Howery. I was stunned!

And thrilled! I was invited to go to Australia to be the 2020 keynote for their national AAC conference. Sadly, COVID veered me from that path, for now. I was sent letters and emails of congratulations on my work from eminent scholars and pioneers in the field of AAC —all because I chose to follow paths that were not necessarily on my roadmap but were provided by a series of fortuitous events. Life is what happens when you are busy making other plans (as musician John Lennon once said), and it can be wondrous if you are open to it.

What inspires me? My inspiration is, and perhaps always has been, to explore and to the degree that I can, understand the fascinating world of communication in all its facets and dimensions. In the fall of 1978, in my Psych 361 class, I sat mesmerized by the video of Ole Ivar Lovaas shaping young Penny's echolalic speech into the word he wanted her to say. I was dazzled by this then, only to be mortified by the results of that approach in my later years. The following year, I took a primate behavior class and followed, with wonder, the approaches of Professors David Premack and Allen and Beatrix Gardner as they explored the communication, learning, and language abilities of our closest animal relations—the great apes. It was those anthropology classes that actually set me on my course to do graduate work in psycholinguistics. In graduate school, I did a research paper on deaf aphasics. It was a time when there was still controversy as to whether sign languages were indeed languages. These studies of deaf people who had had strokes were actually one of the ways the argument was finally settled for the good—sign languages stood the test and were deemed languages indeed.

So, one might ask how has all of this been my inspiration for work in the field of AAC? Well, for all my fascination with communication and language development, I wasn't too interested in the typical path. In 1982, when I was first given the opportunity to work with children and youth with significant disabilities, I was not really constrained by the notion that they needed to talk to communicate. But I did see clearly then, and continue to believe now, that my role was to provide opportunities for them to communicate in other ways, ways that they *could* and ways that, in time and with support, they *would.*

This search, to hear the voices of the voiceless, has been my passion ever since that day. When I attended Harvard Graduate School in the summer of 2007 to learn about universal design for learning from David Rose and Dr. Thomas Hehir, my focus was on communication and the populations of students for whom, in my view, UDL held the greatest promise—children and youth who needed those multiple means of engagement, expression, and representation. It is still on my to-do list to use the UDL guidelines to help people understand AAC and what students with complex communication needs require to be engaged actively and meaningfully in learning and life. Perhaps you may be inspired to engage with me in that endeavor.

My passion for understanding communication continues, both in my research of the lived experience of those who use devices to make their voices heard and in my work-life supporting and teaching others to provide AAC supports and services and learn to listen to the authentic and autonomous voices of all people no matter the mode in which they present it.

The greatest gifts I have obtained on this journey have been the friends, colleagues, and kindred spirits I have gathered along the way. I can happily say I have several friends who use AAC and SGDs in their daily lives. I don't think that would likely have been the case had I not embarked on this path and this inquiry. I can count so many amazing AAC professionals as not only my colleagues but as my friends. I am so blessed by the opportunity to call them up when I have a question about something, to share something exciting I have learned, and to commiserate when the world is not unfolding as it should. I am so grateful that my path has crossed with theirs and that for bits and pieces of the journey we have traveled together.

I also have the gift of continuing my wondering and seeking to understand communication in all its glorious aspects. This, I believe, leads to an understanding of the human spirit and the spirit of all humans to engage in, to quote one wonderful friend I have discovered along the way, *meaning making*[15]. One can learn so much about what it means to be human by connecting meaningfully with those whose lives may be substantively different than ours. To understand the how, we can learn from every being, no matter "abled" or "dis-abled"[16].

---

[15] (Alant 2016)

[16] (Feder Kettay 2019)

Finally, despite myself, I am also able to make a good living doing work that I love and that feeds me so. Not having ever really made any career choices, or life choices, with the goal of making money, I am happy and perhaps a little surprised to say that I am doing just fine financially. Now, that doesn't mean I haven't worked hard at it; I have. And it doesn't mean that I have been lucky enough along the way and in my life circumstances to take risks in this regard. I have never had to worry that I would not be taken care of. But the joy of my life is that I LOVE my work. And my work feeds me figuratively and literally.

Recommendations

Here are a few ideas that have carried me through my career. I hope they will help you feed your joy.

1. Be (wide) open. Be open and attentive to the opportunities that come your way. You may not think of something as an opportunity but if you are open to going in different directions, noticing moments that spark wonder, and taking risks, you can't help but find interesting paths.

2. Listen deeply, intently, and with your whole soul. Listen with a discerning ear, but also a critical ear. Never take what you hear without critical investigation, especially when you are considering someone else's view or understanding of a child. Do your best to listen to the voice of that child, no matter what forms that voice may take.

3. Read on the fringes. Of course, read information in the mainstream as well, but make sure to read authors that are not as widely distributed in the field. Pay attention to what new books and resources are being published and if you can get your hands on as many as you can. You never know what lovely insights and understandings you might glean from discovering a new book on AAC by an author you have yet to read.

4. Make connections. Make connections with others in the field of AAC, but just as importantly, make connections with others who while not in our field, per se, may be able to teach us ways to positively impact the lives of the children we seek to give the affordance of voicing their being in the world. Some of my best learning has come from connection and connecting deeply with those in the fields of vision and those in the field of philosophy.

5. Seek out persons who use AAC in their daily lives as friends and teachers. There is no better teacher than experience, and from sharing their real-life experiences with me, and inviting me into their world, I have not only learned from them, but also have the beginnings of understandings that have served me and those I seek to serve well.

And, lastly, I'll share with you this excerpt from my doctoral dissertation:

How does my grandson work? Why was he placed on this earth this way?

The elderly man held the boy on his lap. There was a typewriter in front of them. The elderly man wondered "what can this boy do? How can I share my thoughts with him and he with me? How does this boy work?"

The boy was no prize human being. He wriggled around and uncomfortably flailed his arms with abandon. The boy drooled too, even though he was well past the age of learning to swallow.

The boy liked to bang on the downstairs piano and make a jumble of sounds until somebody moved him out of the range of the keys. He often visited the office and seemed interested in his typewriter. The boy started touching the keys of the typewriter. The boy noticed that they would go down if he hit them and sometimes this left a little mark on the paper in the typewriter.[17]

Michael Williams, a prominent writer in the field of AAC, who himself uses a SGD among other things to communicate, shares this story as his introduction to written communication on the knee of his grandfather. I share it as a lovely example of a caring grandfather who is acting with pedagogical tact as he seeks ways of authentically understanding the child before him. Who is this child? How does this child work? How can I come to know him? How can we come to know each other? These are the questions that are guiding the grandfather as he places the child before the machine. Following the child's lead, and attending to his abilities in other areas (the

---

[17] (Howard C. Shane, et al. 2012)

playing of the piano) the elderly man takes the child onto his knee and provides the opportunity for access and for exploration.[18]

I share this as my wish for you. I hope you can channel Michael's grandfather in your interactions with every child, especially those who some may consider "no prize human beings." We are each an amazingly prized human being, seeking ways to let each child's voice and prizes shine forth.

Ways to Connect with Me

Email: khowery@ualberta.ca

Email: kateconsulting@icloud.com

Facebook: Kathy Look Howery

Twitter: @klhowery

Kathy Howery began her career nearly 40 years ago focused on finding ways for students with the most complex needs to share their voices in the world. Her research focuses on using phenomenological methods to explore the lived experience of young people who speak with (or through) speech generating devices. She provides ongoing consultation to Alberta school jurisdictions, has developed an online certificate for teaching students with complex communication needs (CCN), and is a member of the Alberta Low Incidence Collaborative Supports team with primary responsibility in the area of CCN.

[18] (Howery 2017)

Some Things I Cannot Change, But Until I Try, I'll Never Know

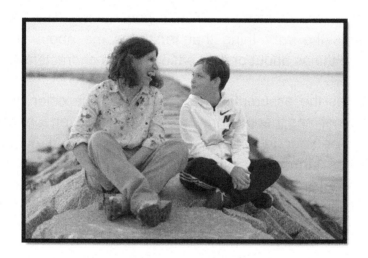

India Ochs

Photo by Kelly Eskelsen Photography

* * *

The 19th century showman P.T. Barnum once said, "No one ever made a difference by being like everyone else." [19]

I have never fit in any stereotype or anyone's perception of who they think I am, and this book makes that point. Wait. Did

---

[19] *The Greatest Showman*, 2017

I just refer to this book when this chapter is supposed to be a snapshot of me? Have the publishers allowed me to break protocol and talk about the process of writing this chapter?

When the coauthors were invited to participate in this book, we were encouraged to write about the challenges we faced, what inspires us, how we created and grew our disability offering, and other topics related to the augmentative and alternative communication (AAC) community. This format represents the very thing that frustrates me about society: assuming things about people based on one characteristic.

Sometimes the assumptions are based on the color of your skin. Sometimes people draw conclusions based on where you live or your job, or, in this case, having a disability. Sometimes those assumptions stem from a general (mis)perception of how people react to things. Generally, one needs to understand that it's not what a person says or even the intent that matters; it's how the other person perceives the message.

Two things glaringly jumped out when we were provided writing prompts to help outline each section. First, words like "creating and growing your disability offering" and "your personal experience with" or "in the disability space" irked me. Yes, I have a speech disability, and yes, this is a book about leaders connected to the AAC world, but my disability has never been part of my life. Don't get me wrong, I fully acknowledge that my disability will always be with me, 24/7— for my whole life, but it has never defined me nor been the focus of my life's work.

The second thing that sparked dismay was the description for this opening section. It was (is) supposed to focus on a challenge that impacted our lives, which would be all well and good for me, as someone who thrives on challenges; but, the words included in the prompt, "a pivotal moment when you deeply questioned your ability to keep moving forward..." caught my attention. I feel this does not apply to me. I have never once questioned my ability to move on—from anything. It has always annoyed me when people assume everyone struggles with loss or obstacles (or the appearance of obstacles).

As I read the chapter's expected format, I thought, "Once again, I don't fit in. I am going to have to go against the grain yet another time." That said, I was not going to walk away from this book just because I may not like the question asked or the way the suggested prompt was written.

I racked my mind trying to think of any point in my life when I even came close to questioning myself or what I was doing. Those who get to know me quickly see how scary the extent of my memory can be. I easily can share detailed accounts of stories all the way back to age two, not to mention I recount stories about others, ones they themselves may have forgotten. But still, I had no memory of a challenge that questioned my abilities.

The closest incident I could think of was way back in third grade, which would have been the 1983-84 school year. I was at church one Sunday filled with excitement because I was finally old enough to join the children's choir.

By nature, I am an off-the-cuff kind of person who will do things in the moment (four-day fall break road trip randomly heading west, anyone?). At the same time, if my instincts tell me there is something I want, either now or in the future, I tend to stick to it. It's why I never wavered from wanting to be an attorney from the age of five, deciding on the name of my firstborn son at age ten, or yearning to turn age 18 so that I could finally vote. Wanting to be in my church's choir was no different.

There was nothing special about my church at the time. It was just a normal Methodist church set out in the country, with a large hill to roll down and an outside cathedral area in the far-left corner of the acreage that sparked excitement in kids who liked anything outside of the routine services. But it was my church, my family at the time, and so on that Sunday, I sat in the pew repeatedly checking the program in anticipation of the time when kids were allowed to leave the service to go downstairs. When that moment arrived, I quickly got up, trying to walk fast to the back of the sanctuary without causing too much of a scene as I passed by all the stained-glass windows within the bright white walls. I ran down the stairs, through the all-purpose room used for meals and other gatherings, and into the annex where the younger kids had Sunday school. The area was divided by old, brown, folding wall partitions to create different spaces for different activities.

When I arrived at the partition, I heard the female choir director talking to the kids. I froze. At that moment, I thought to myself, "I want this so bad, but will they actually let me join with my speech disability?" It was a rare moment in my life when tears started to well up and stream down my cheeks. I cannot remember exactly how long I just stood there—unable to open the partition yet refusing to leave—but it felt like an eternity. And that is representative of who I am. Yes, I froze in that moment, not knowing how to approach the director or how to tell her I wanted to join the choir. Yet, I WANTED to be in the choir, and I was never going to just walk away from what I wanted, simply because I got scared in that moment of being accepted into something. Eventually, the choir director saw me standing outside of the partition and invited me in. After I calmed down and explained that I was there to join the choir, she welcomed me with no reservations.

Almost four decades and many challenges later, not much has changed. Let me rephrase that last part. I say many challenges, but the reality is most of the "challenges" in my life did not come from my inability to do something. The challenges often stem from societal norms that, at best, overlook, and, at worst, blatantly discriminate against certain demographics.

Take, for instance, how I was invited to more than 80 in-person interviews while job hunting in 2006, and how I was called in for more than 80 interviews a few years later in 2011 when I was looking for another job.

I applied for jobs in a variety of places, including government, nonprofit, law firms, and legal-based, policy-based, and human rights-based organizations. I knew I was highly qualified for basically every job I applied for. But, like virtually any job, most employers don't consider every single application that comes in, especially if these employers receive hundreds of applications for a position. Honestly, I wasn't expecting to actually get so many interview requests. In a lot of ways, though, the large volume of interviews motivated me and reinforced my feeling of knowing I was qualified and deserved the job. Time after time, my resume and/or cover letter reflected my qualifications for the position and what potentially would set me apart from other applicants.

The fact that it took more than 80 interviews—on two different occasions—to finally get an offer is not simply a sign of a competitive job market. I believe it is also a sign of the fear and ignorance many in society still have when interacting with someone with a speech disability.

In some ways, I was prepared for these kinds of interactions, not only from past interviews, but from life in general. I have seen how some strangers react around me. How I respond to this really does depend on the moment. Certain times, I knew it was worth being aggressive to try to prove why they wanted to interview me in the first place, such as at a legal aid office I had clerked at during law school. Other times, I knew it wasn't worth pushing when I saw I was getting completely shut down in the interview after one or two follow-up questions, and it was hard to keep the conversation moving. I also will say 98% of the time I never even mention my disability going into the interview, but I have always done as much background research as possible on the people interviewing me, if I knew who they would be. And, if I thought it was appropriate, I would bring copies of two or three articles profiling me to show the disability didn't impact my work. Luckily, I am a quick judge of people and my instincts are almost always right, so I knew how to respond to questions and dynamics from all kinds of people.

However, many times, I could see that sense of fear from the interviewer within the first minute of my interview, whether it was through body language, a change of tone, the way they suddenly rephrased questions or kept the interview short. Yet, the fact that I went on that many interviews also is proof of how rejection never slowed me down from seeking employment.

The same is true in the aftermath of running a political campaign.

Days before writing this chapter, I lost my election for a seat on my county's board of education. It was the first time my district had ever elected someone to the board of education, and a lot factored into this strange election, in the midst of the COVID-19 pandemic, but at the end of the day, I lost. Did I like that I lost? Of course not. Yet, it is what it is. I had done everything I could, with the resources I had, and in the setting at the time.

What I disliked more goes with the theme of this section: people assumed I would be upset. I did not say anything out loud because I did not want to undermine the sympathy (empathy?) and compassion people had for me when expressing words of encouragement. But between you and me (and all the other readers of this book), it became frustrating to continually hear words like, "You will regroup from this." or "You will find a way to transition." or "You will come out of this fine."

Again, that is not who I am. By nature, I don't regroup or transition from a loss because I don't dwell on the negative. It was an election, and I believe I, far and wide, deserved to win, but I didn't, and there is nothing I can do about it. It's not the end of the world, and anyone who knows me, knows I don't walk away from anything or anyone I am invested in. Win or lose, there is never going to be a break from advocating for our kids and teachers in our public schools. We learn from the past and get stronger from it, but there was never a reason for me to dwell on it or take time to mourn. Again, it was just an election. I am still alive. I was not even knocked down, per say. I still have things to do in life.

These instances reminded me of the climactic scene in *Captain Marvel* when Carol Danvers is going against the Supreme Being for the last time. Danvers was told that she had been saved from being a human, implying that she had been weak when on Earth, but in that moment, Danvers says with confidence, "You're right. I'm only human."[20] She then replays the flashbacks from her past when she had been knocked down as a kid or in boot camp, finally seeing how she got back up each time, and kept going. In the comic book Danvers is quoted as saying "But being the best you can be…That's doable. That's possible for anybody if they put their mind to it."[21] I have always shared that mindset, despite any assumptions about my abilities and my character society might throw my way.

---

[20] Carol Danvers (Earth-616)

https://marvel.fandom.com/wiki/Carol_Danvers_(Earth-616)

[21] *Ms. Marvel Volume 2 #50*

My inspiration, my motivation for all that I do in life is rooted in a simple goal: to support those around me.

From the very beginning, my calling to be an attorney was based on a desire to: (1) help people find their self-confidence, (2) make sure they knew their rights, and (3) make sure their voices were heard.

That philosophy has never differed throughout all my jobs and running for local office. Law and policy are in my blood, but being an attorney always meant more than only being in court (as much as my heart sped up with joy when stepping into a courtroom).

To me, becoming an attorney meant being a storyteller and a counselor, a defender and a cheerleader, an investigator and an advocate, a voice for the people, and a foundation to get everyone's voices heard. I have always believed that it is critical to know who we are interacting with, which is why taking time to listen to another person is so important in every area of life.

When applying for a new job, I often include in my cover letter how important it is to understand how our work impacts those we work for and with. I discuss how what may become routine or daily work to us can be new and life-changing to our clients or others with whom we engage.

Since my early 20s, I wished all law school students could spend 24 hours in jail just for a glimpse of what it was like so that they would have a better concept of what their clients might face. In the same way patients will tune out a doctor as soon as they hear a bad diagnosis, clients who have been in jail overnight are less likely to listen to their attorney given how emotionally shaken they are.

These scenarios can be applied to any situation, which is why I have always believed in taking the time to talk to—and listen to—the other person first, before trying to relay a message or get a job done. The ability to learn who someone is, to show them respect and let them know I am listening, is what has helped me find success in all that I do, whether professionally when running a nonprofit, as a human rights attorney, or personally as a parent talking to a group of four-year-old kids or supporting fellow families as PTA president.

Public service and changing things from within the system have been part of my motivation in all that I do, for as long as I can remember. Growing up, I was taken to many protests and surrounded by people assisting families from lower socio-economic communities. I saw the need to help others but also saw how change could be more effective from within the system versus fighting the system. Also, my love for the United States was so strong that I had posters of George Washington and Thomas Jefferson on my wall as a kid, instead of Michael Jackson or Kirk Cameron.

If you combine that passion to serve my country and its people, through law and advocacy, it becomes easy to see why I did everything from serving in AmeriCorps after law school to working at national nonprofits on human rights and juvenile justice initiatives, to working for the federal government and volunteering in the US Coast Guard Auxiliary, to actively supporting my community on education and racial justice issues.

I struggle with the concept of what I personally have gained from my work, or, I should say, from my life's work. Essentially, I do not look for any self-gain in anything I do. I approach life with the thought that I am only happy if you are happy. If my son says, "Have a good day." as he leaves for school, my usual response is "Only if you do." I definitely do not want to put pressure on others to have a good day if they can't or don't want to, but it's my nature to want others to be safe and successful every day.

I also am not the kind of person who needs to hear "thank you" or "congratulations." Yes, I appreciate it when given, but any personality test will show I am much more inclined to thrive in a hurricane than with praise. That said, it does give me tremendous pleasure when I see I made a difference or helped someone find the self-motivation they had hidden away within them.

I still remember two instances as a summer law clerk at Maryland's Legal Aid Bureau, which seemed par for the course to me, but apparently was not for the attorneys I worked for. In one instance, I was assigned a case with a six-year-old girl seeking Social Security Disability Insurance (SSDI) benefits. It made me smile that I was able to successfully take the case to administrative court after four senior attorneys had passed over the case when not finding enough evidence to even take it to court. Yet, what really stood out was when I was called into the supervising attorney's office after I submitted the written brief prior to the administrative hearing. According to the attorney, the mother of the client had called her, in tears, saying she had just read the brief and it was the first time anyone had been able to truly capture what her daughter's needs were. The attorney also said she had never had a client call crying in tears of happiness before. While I appreciated that moment, I thought to myself, "I am just doing my job."

Along the same lines, I accompanied an attorney to court on another case I had helped prepare. Prior to entering the courtroom, I simply chatted with the client as we waited on a bench. Afterward, as we left court, the client gave me a hug. On the way back to the office, the attorney commented how she had never gotten a hug from any client, ever. Again, I thought I hadn't done anything out of the ordinary in my work or in interacting with the client—at least nothing out of the ordinary in the way I do things. However, I appreciated the fact that we not only had won the case, but that I made an impact in a way not everyone apparently does.

My campaign for the board of education also produced similar instances of showing that what I was doing mattered. Several people commented that I was the only person on the ballot they had total confidence in. One of those voters, who was a parent in her 30s, shared how it was her first time ever voting, and that she only did it to vote for me. I also got emails from parents of children with disabilities, who expressed not only how they were motivated by me but were also counting on me. One parent shared that her 19-year-old autistic son had voted in the primary for the first time, taking the time to learn about all five candidates, and deciding that I was the best choice. Those kinds of messages confirmed that both my advocacy and campaign for office were making a difference, regardless of the outcome in November.

Recommendations

1. Listen to your gut. If you want to be successful, it's just this simple: Know what you are doing. Love what you are doing. And believe in what you are doing.

2. Keep on moving. Even if you are on the right track, you'll get run over if you just sit there.

3. Learn from, but don't dwell, on whatever happens. Don't let yesterday take up too much of today.

4. Don't walk away. The best way out of difficulty is through it.

5. Stay proud of yourself and what you do. Live in such a way that you would not be ashamed to sell your parrot to the town gossip.

My hope for you is what I hope for everyone: Don't lose your passion for what you love and never stop going after what you envision as success.

Never let others set the bar for you or attempt to define who you are. It is fine to ask for advice or assistance, but only if you want it, and if you accept it based on who you are and who you want to be.

There are very few motivational songs from musicals that don't cause the hairs on my arms to stand up and make me want to jump up and fight the fight. And it's a no-brainer that "*The Impossible Dream* (The Quest)" from *Man of La Mancha* is one of them, especially when you hear performances in a booming voice filled with passion. It's worthwhile to share some analysis when breaking down the lyrics.

As in its name, the song starts with the line "To dream the impossible dream." But is any dream really impossible? I don't think so, if you truly believe in it. You still may never achieve a dream for dozens of reasons, but it does not mean the dream is impossible to go after.

The same is true of the lyrics "This is my quest, to follow that star, no matter how hopeless, no matter how far." Again, I don't see a reason why following any star would be hopeless, if it is your quest.

Later on, it says "To run where the brave dare not go. To right the unrightable wrong," and "To fight for the right, without question or pause." Those words illustrate what my own life's work has always been about. Hopefully, you share in that ability to run where others dare not go, regardless of where that "where" is for you.

The final lyrics I want to comment on are, "And the world will be better for this, that one man, scorned and covered with scars, still strove with his last ounce of courage, to reach the unreachable star." Those words go back to my original message at the start of this chapter: Regardless of what society might throw at you, despite the challenges you might face along the way, and the numerous times you might get knocked down, keep getting up. Keep going after what you believe in. And when you do that, the world will be a better place because of the impact your actions have on those you know and don't know.

My Community

Watch my interview with Mai Ling Chan on Cognixion's What's New? What's Next? in AAC:

Ways to Connect with Me

Email: india.ochs@gmail.com

LinkedIn:@indiaochs

Facebook: @indiaochs

India Ochs, currently employed by the U.S. government, has been involved in advocacy issues for more than 30 years. Previously, India was a senior project associate at the Pretrial Justice Institute, working on juvenile detention reform issues, and the legal officer for the Robert F. Kennedy Memorial

Center for Human Rights, during which time she developed and coordinated legal and legislative initiatives with human rights activists on the ground in 24 countries. India is an experienced public speaker with extensive work in organizing, facilitating, and participating in leadership workshops and conferences. Licensed to practice law, India has a JD with a certificate in family law & social policy from Syracuse University College of Law, and a master's degree in public affairs with a certificate in nonprofit management from UNC Greensboro.

Taking a Stand for Learners with Complex Communication Needs

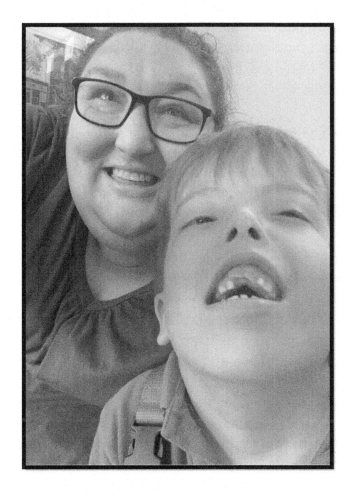

Kate Ahern, MSEd

Becoming an Exceptional AAC Leader

* * *

I've never really felt like I fit in. For a lot of my early life, it was one of the things I wanted most—close friends, to belong.

Around the time I started high school, someone suggested I volunteer in the special education classroom. So, I started spending my free periods helping out. My home life wasn't great. I struggled with friendships. Those periods of volunteer work were a highlight of my day. I felt like I belonged in that classroom. I enjoyed the company of the students and they enjoyed mine.

There was one student who was nonspeaking. He was my age and communicated by pointing to picture symbols attached to his wheelchair tray. We liked hanging out together, and eventually I started working for him at his home as a personal care attendant.

Coming from a modest size suburb, I also ended up working at a local day camp for students with more significant disabilities and seeing him there, too. That led to me volunteering at a camp for children with muscular dystrophy. At that camp, I also gravitated toward the couple of children who used augmentative and alternative communication (AAC).

As a result, by 1994, at the age of 17, I had already had personal AAC experience with both nonelectronic communication boards and books and with two different electronic communication systems, the LightTalker by PRC and the original DynaVox. Additionally, during my last year of high school, I took American Sign Language at a local community college. I didn't precisely know what to call it, but I already knew I wanted to work with children who had complex communication needs.

When it was time to select a college, I wanted three things. First, I wanted to be able to major in special education. Second, I wanted a small women's college; at that time, women with leadership roles in government and business were graduates of women's colleges and though I didn't see myself in government or business, I believed there had to be something to the skillset gained at a women's college that would help me. Finally, I needed scholarships or grants. In the end, Simmons College (now Simmons University) in Boston met all my criteria. Another thing I found at Simmons was a place where I belonged, at least some of the time.

As per Massachusetts law, I was required to double major to be eligible for a special education teacher's license, the idea being that a math teacher will major in math and in high school education. Of course, being a special education major gave no obvious double major, but I found I loved sociology.

It was a good thing I found a place in the sociology department, because the education department, especially the special education department, frowned on just about every part of my existence. I was an out lesbian, a work-study/scholarship student, and, for the most part, a big mouth. I didn't mean to be a big mouth, it was just that when I saw injustice, my mouth started going.

The head of the special education department made it clear that I was not acceptable by her standards. In one memorable example, I requested that an expensive textbook we were required to purchase and read only one chapter of, be put on reserve in the library. The director very publicly shamed me, saying that purchasing books was part of the requirement of being a college student; if I couldn't do that I didn't belong there. Then, an hour or so later, she pulled me aside and gave me a copy of the book, she had three. She could have easily put that copy on reserve, so it was clear to me that shaming me for not having financial resources was actually her primary goal.

Luckily, just after this happened, the college hired a new assistant professor, Susan Ainsleigh, to cover most of the intensive (now known as severe) special education program. When she was hired, she was told that I was her *problem*. She turned out to be a wonderful mentor and we are still friends to this day.

Between Susan and my advisor in the sociology department, Ellen Borges, I had guideposts to help me finish the five-year combined bachelor's plus master's degree program with a 4.0 GPA and a job offer. My experience at Simmons College was rocky, though at times wonderful. My queerness, financial situation, big mouth, and the fact that I still seemed to not fit in, a lot of the time, were ongoing issues. Yet, I was exceptionally well prepared both as a teacher and to think critically about society and the world.

Moving into the world of work wasn't any easier than high school or college. I adored teaching, relished my work with my students teaching communication, and implementing AAC and assistive technology. The times were different then, there was no focus on literacy or numeracy for those with intensive special needs. I regret that I didn't know better back then. I taught how I was trained to teach but, in retrospect, there was so much more I could have and should have done.

The larger issue for me was that I was perfectly happy to talk about teaching my students and supporting AAC around the clock. I loved what I was doing so much that I talked about little else. I didn't fit in with teachers who wanted to go for drinks or have Tupperware parties. Add to that, my drive for social justice and my trouble with being tactful when things were unjust, and I didn't make friends at work. I could not understand why I was rated both an excellent teacher and a poor employee. To me, my sole purpose was to educate my students. I didn't grasp all of the other things that were unspoken yet expected of me. There had been no coursework in *making nice* with administrators, paraprofessionals, and hordes of auxiliary professionals and therapists. I was terrible at *playing the game.*

Around this time, things also went haywire, or more haywire, in my family life. My younger sister, Stacey, had been in and out of mental health facilities for her bipolar syndrome and post-traumatic disorder since she was 14 years old, about when I left for college. At age 21, she tried to take her own life. It wasn't the first time she had done this, but it was certainly the most serious attempt to date. She took large quantities of her prescribed medication and was having continuous seizures. Eventually, she was put in a helicopter to transfer to a hospital in Boston. It was a rough few weeks while she was in the ICU, on dialysis, in a medically induced coma, and the staff worked to keep her alive. My brother, Brendan, also a special education teacher, flew home from Hawaii where he lived. When she eventually stepped down from ICU to a floor unit, she had a feeding tube placed and, although she could kick and scream, she could not speak or use her arms.

About six weeks later she was ready to be moved to a rehabilitation facility. We were unaware that she was hallucinating at this time and she screamed continuously. Her thrashing caused her hair to matte and eventually someone shaved the back of her head. After some time in rehab, she gained the ability to point with a large marker taped closed as a stylus. She was able to progress to communicating by spelling on a board. She didn't like the communication boards the hospital gave her, finding them insulting since they had picture symbols. I used the communication software in my classroom to make her a book; I also built a handle for the book because she had trouble holding it.

One day when I went to visit, Stacey told me, by pointing to letters and words in her book, that the previous night she pressed the call light because she needed the restroom. The aide came in, shut off the call light, and left. My sister pressed it again, the aide shut it off again. By the third repeat of this Stacey started to scream. It was really the only option she had to communicate. Despite big signs I had made and posted explaining her communication book, it wasn't offered. So, she screamed. The aide came back again and slapped her across the face, twice. The next day she had the bruise to prove it. We were able to file the incident with the hospital, but I am not sure what happened in the end. Perhaps the aide was let go or perhaps she was just moved to a different floor. That experience changed me.

Abuse prevention became one of my priorities with my students from then on. They needed to know what was acceptable and what wasn't, and they needed to have the communication skills to be accurate reporters if something happened. Though it wasn't easy to phrase, they also needed the self-regulation skills to avoid resorting to screaming, aggression or other "maladaptive behaviors" that could trigger unstable workers— workers who might hurt them. Of course, abuse is always the fault of the abuser, but I wanted to keep my students as safe as possible.

Eventually, my sister graduated from rehab and began a long process of accepting her new disabilities from her brain injury and making a life for herself. She did speak again; in fact, her first words were, "thank you" when I finished shaving her legs. I have to say, trusting me to shave her legs was a huge leap of   faith!
I changed jobs about a year after Stacey's brain injury. For the next eight years I worked at, what is called in Massachusetts, a collaborative program. It is basically a program where school districts pool their funding to educate those with low-incidence disabilities. I was a classroom teacher and the coordinator (day-to-day operations director) of a summer camp for children with complex disabilities. My students were amazing. I loved teaching them and my class grew because of the great results we were getting. Although our agency capped classes at seven to eight students, my class was regularly over ten and once reached 13 students. About half of my students used AAC.

I immersed myself in learning about AAC and assistive technology for learners with complex communication and other needs. I read articles, researched at the library, borrowed devices to try them out, and essentially spent the time I wasn't teaching, writing evaluations, individualized education programs (IEPs), or preparing lessons learning about AAC. I learned about the AAC communication competencies and tried to embed them into all my lessons. I still struggled with *playing the game* with colleagues and administration. I just didn't know how to keep all of the adults happy and maintain positive relationships with everyone. Some days things were great, and other days, I seemed to have upset people and never really knew why. Things weren't always easy, but I loved my work, and I loved my students.

Part of the problem seemed to be that my colleagues found me to be a know-it-all. I talked too much about work and with too much conviction. To take some pressure off myself, I started a blog, *Teaching Learners with Multiple Special Needs*, offering resources to other intensive special needs teachers. Over time, it became a very popular and award-winning blog. My focus was always on content. I hadn't heard the expression, *content is king*, but I certainly lived by it. I wrote content that I would find useful myself. The blog let me talk about teaching special education and AAC as much as I wanted to; it was a great option and it helped others. A win-win.

Then in 2008, my sister attempted to end her life again. It was eight years after the attempt causing her initial brain injuries and, in that time, she had learned how to walk and speak again, although using her arms and hands was much more difficult and she never was able to write by hand or drive a car again. She was also less than a month away from a bachelor's degree in creative writing from Sarah Lawrence College. This time, the damage from the suicide attempt was far too severe. After time spent in a coma on life support, my father, brother (who had flown in from Hawaii), and I were there when she was removed from the ventilator. She died surrounded by love.

Grief took me down, hard. I was devastated. My entire world seemed black. At work, I somehow managed to turn everyone, except my students and their parents, against me. Part of that was my grief, part of it was the stigma of losing a sibling to suicide (everyone assumed I must be mentally ill as well), and part of it was beyond my comprehension. I entered a period of my life when I felt lost and like I was surrounded by darkness. With extreme difficulty I found a new teaching job, where I only stayed for a few years. Then I took a job with a nonprofit as an assistive technology consultant. Again, I only lasted for a few years. At the teaching job, they took issue with my blog, despite conversations before hiring me where they made clear that they would allow me to continue writing it. At the nonprofit job, I was often put in positions to do work I really didn't feel qualified for, work with children with high incidence disabilities, and with adults with a wide variety of disabilities. During that time though, I was able to build a reputation as a local, regional, and national public speaker about learners with complex communication needs. I discovered I loved public speaking almost as much as I liked working directly with my students. Eventually, I struck out on my own and started a private practice.

I initially worried about attracting enough business to be financially solvent, but my friends assured me that wouldn't be a concern. I was scared, yet thrilled to go out on my own. Money was very tight, but the work was on my own terms and the needs of my students could always come first. I never had to assure some administrator that what I was doing was worth it. I never had to justify to colleagues that my efforts weren't going to make them look bad. I never had to grit my teeth as another professional treated my student with disregard or disrespect. Going out on my own also allowed me to address one of the most unmet needs in working with children who use AAC: teaching their families.

Things haven't been perfect in my professional life or personal life since I opened my private practice, AAC Voices. My ability to turn people off without knowing what I said or did still shows up at times.

In addition, my brother, Brendan, ended his life with a deliberate heroin overdose in 2018, ten years after my sister, and I was thrown back into the peculiar grief of sibling suicide loss.

Some time later came COVID-19, as did opening an online school for children and young adults who use AAC. Serving more than 100 students from many states and countries, the online school has been a massive success. It will continue after the pandemic as the Brendan and Stacey Ahern Academy Cooperative with a focus on educating homeschool students who use AAC.

Recommendations

1. Do the next right thing.

2. Trust the process.

3. Just keep going.

4. Follow your own path and be true to yourself.

My Community

Watch my interview with Mai Ling Chan on Cognixion's What's New? What's Next? in AAC:

Ways to Connect with Me

Please visit www.AACvoices.org for more information about my practice or to reach me.

Kate Ahern is an educational specialist in complex communication needs in private practice. She is certified as an intensive special needs teacher for ages birth through adult in Massachusetts. Kate has vast experience in the field of assistive technology with children and young adults.

A Reluctant Public Advocate Shines in the Spotlight

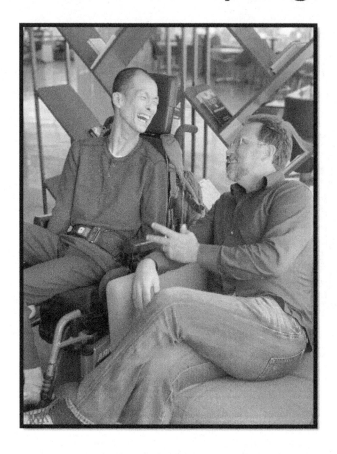

Tim Jin

Photo by Mai Ling Chan

* * *

I was born with cerebral palsy and couldn't use my hands, walk, or talk like a normal baby and toddler. I was my parents' first born and was conceived in the mid- 1970s. My family is from South Korea and my parents had recently arrived in America. Like a rookie, waiting for their first pitch, my "eomma" and "appa" were eagerly waiting to hit a grand slam out of the park, but as soon as I was born, they felt that they struck out with their first child. Instead of leaving me behind, like an old pair of shoes that you crunch the heels in the back and use them as outdoor slippers that you drag around and don't care about, my parents decided to take me home and raise me as best as they could.

My biggest challenge in life has always been communicating with my parents.

With no way of communicating with me, I feel that my mom needed to separate herself, as a new mom, from me. I don't really have fond memories of my mom when I was a baby. Maybe it is because my parents needed to adjust to a new country and had to struggle to provide for the family, or maybe my mom thought that she had failed to give a perfect infant to the family's name, but a lot of my memories were with my grandma. She always kissed my feet after I got off the bus from school as I was in the wheelchair, dangling my legs as if I was playing on a swing set. I was my grandma's pride and joy, and without her inspiration in my parents' lives, maybe my mom and dad would have thought twice about putting me in the crib in their house? I will never know and will never ask my parents. Some things are meant to be a layer in the dust and never be polished again.

My grandma was a very religious lady. She thought that God would save me and heal me, magically give me the perfect body, make me be straight as a flagpole, and not flopping around like undercooked bacon. My parents used to take me to these prayer meetings at church where they would pray for me, and I've been laid down many times by the holy hands of church evangelists, claiming that they had the power of God. But my parents put me to bed, and the next morning their prayers weren't answered because I was still the same. The same defective child.

By this time, I was putting words together in my speech and developing as a normal child, like my two younger brothers, and we played and fought like siblings do. This is where my folks saw my spark and when my mom and I became closer. To this day, my mom and my family are my biggest fans, but they will probably never read this chapter. My parents gave me and my brothers their attention equally, and I think that is why my brothers and I still remain close, even after our midlife crisis stages.

Throughout my childhood, I've had countless speech therapy sessions. I can't tell you how much speech-language pathology, physical therapy and occupational therapy I've had. But instead of therapy, my parents chose to rely on their faith and sought out science and treatments they thought would make me prosper. I can remember when my speech therapist caught me swearing in the hallway in school and said something like, "our sessions are definitely working" or something like that. Even to this day, when I am speaking from my natural voice, I always remember to pronounce my words correctly, making sure I enunciate "/k/, /ed/, /se/, and /s/" at the end of each word.

I've had many augmentative and alternative (AAC) devices in my life. I've been using my feet to write for as long as I can remember, and when I learned how to spell my name in elementary school, I learned how to type everything I wanted to on a typewriter. The keyboard has become an appendix to my body. If I'm in the zone, I can type on my computer without looking, and I never liked any kind of word prediction on a desktop because it slows me down causing me to lose my thought.

My first alternative augmentative communication device was a Handivoice. The best way to describe the device is like those Speak and Spell toys, but like five times bigger. I was using the device before I turned ten. I needed to spell every word phonetically. It drove my parents and teachers bonkers because I went to class to learn how to spell correctly, and then I went to my speech therapists and they would teach me how to use the Handivoice by sounding out the words. Even to this day, my spelling is not the greatest. Good thing for autocorrect.

In high school, I had a twenty-pound laptop that I would carry around with me all time in between classes. It was also an alternative augmentative communication device with text-to-speech output. I had the same setup as Stephen Hawking at the time. I've had so many devices in my life, it's almost impossible to keep track. My family always supported my AAC needs. You wouldn't let your child wear the same shoes as their feet grow, so why would you let someone use the same device for their entire life and not improve their communication skills? Currently, I've been using an iPad Pro and use many different AAC apps to talk. I also do consulting with many companies to test their apps and find ways for improvements. They consider me a power user.

My voice became vibrant to my parents as soon as I got my first AAC device. My vocal cords started to come from a computer instead of from my mouth. But because of the language barrier between me and my parents, it is much easier for me to speak to them in Korean and English combined together along with my speech rhythm from my cerebral palsy, but even still, my mom and dad have a hard time understanding me unless we are in the same room. No matter how technology improves with AAC, I will always have a hard time communicating with my parents because of my disability and the language barriers. Sometimes, I am sad knowing that the wonderful couple who gave birth to me will never truly know their first born, and maybe that is why I love my brothers differently than mom and dad. They understand— there are no barriers between us.

I have never envied my brothers because they are able-bodied. I can't speak for them, but having a sibling who is disabled, their prospective role in the family is different. Even though I'm the oldest of three sons, my two brothers have always been a shield for me when we were growing up. Not like being overprotective, but they notice things that I still don't see or choose to ignore, like how people react to me when we are hanging out together. For example, when we are at a restaurant, they notice things like I don't get my own menu, or the waiter talks to them and not to me, asking, "what does he want," as if I'm not there. Because I get this a lot when I'm out and about, I don't see these things at all. It's like my senses and awareness of other people have been camouflaged over time.

I also see my brothers and my sisters-in-law teaching the same awareness to my nieces and that makes me happy. I often let my brothers know that their daughters (seven of them) are the best gift they ever gave me. Being an uncle to my Jinsters, my nickname for them, is what I look forward to on birthdays, holidays, and random other days when we check in on each other. There is nothing like seeing them growing up and being their favorite uncle. I can't wait for them to get older and bring home potential loves of their life so I can drill their mates.

Even though I'm disabled, I never liked being in the spotlight. I know that a lot of people who have seen me before, heard my presentations, or are my friends, see me as an inspiration. Just because I can do certain things with my feet, I've never seen myself being a role model to anyone. The thought has never come to me that I should inspire other people through my actions or words. Being in the spotlight all the time was never my intention but is the result of being on several boards of directors, committees, speaking engagements and nonprofit work. Although I like to broadcast what I'm doing most of the time and advocate in and for the disabled community, it doesn't mean that I like to be in the spotlight all the time. Actually, my comfort zone is behind the curtain, rolling as fast as I can on the hamster wheel. But, because of my personality, I attract a wide range of people if they are willing to be patient with me and wait for me to communicate using my AAC device.

My purpose in being a self-advocate and an AAC user is not for personal gain or to educate people either. If the audience sees me as their role model, that is not my goal. There are two kinds of people in this world. Some people like to just float around and have a good time and when they see a giant wave coming, they immediately head for the shores. Then, you have people like myself, who always has to have the glass full to the brim and ready to spill over. I was taught by my parents to give everything my best. I either have to dive into a project or don't do it at all. I'm either all in, or all out. I am never somewhere in the middle, waiting to be called on.

This sometimes hurts me at the end of the day because I take on a lot. I am always doing something and feel overwhelmed most of the time, but this is my normal state. I never look back at what I have accomplished. I'm always looking ahead to the future. There is no reason for me to dwell on the past because it's a total waste of time. I also believe that because of my mindset, I have had more opportunities than I could've imagined. More avenues have opened up for me when I accepted that I can't live in the past.

As a child, I was always in the media, either in print, or some Korean tv channels doing a half-hour special on me because they didn't know anyone who could use their feet like I do. In some ways, I felt like a circus act, where everyone was staring at me and wondering what I was going to do next. Because of people's awkwardness with me, I usually take the initiative to go up to them first and break the ice. I also use a lot of humor when I'm speaking to break the tension in the room. Once people are able to overlook my wheelchair, feet, and spasticity, I can quickly make friends with almost anyone. I like to joke around with my brothers and say that when it's my time to pass this life, they will need to rent an auditorium for all the people who will come, and that the food bill after the service will probably be just as much as college tuition for my nieces. I've never had any problem talking to strangers and making friends.

For those who can't or don't know how to overlook my disability and treat me as if I'm at the dentist picking out a toy after an appointment, I usually ignore them altogether. I've learned you can't be friends with everyone you meet, and I don't waste my time with people who are going to treat me like a child.

Because I am who I am and just don't care what others think of me, I've always been confident in whatever I set my mind to, and I have always been very independent and responsible. I am also proud of my financial independence and ability to manage money. My credit score is better than most people because I can handle my responsibilities and don't have codependency issues.

For my 38th birthday, I wanted to go skydiving. It took me months to find a place that would let me jump out of a perfectly good airplane. I finally found a local skydiving school nearby that catered to people with disabilities, and my doctor signed off that I was good to go for my very first tandem jump. I had already been working out every day in the gym to have better strength and flexibility and was ready to go. But when I got to the skydiving place and they saw my cerebral palsy, the head instructor said it would be too dangerous to take me up and jump with me. I ended up finding a different skydiving school and instructors who didn't question my abilities. If you're wondering if I ended up falling from the sky, there is a clip of it on YouTube. Freefalling is the best feeling I have ever felt, and I wanted to experience more of the freefall than the parachute opening.

I'm so glad I was able to complete that goal because I've also had many disappointments in my life. After a while these things become demons, eating away at me, and I start to doubt myself and I lose hope. It takes a lot for me to lose momentum, and I've always found a way to get that spark back because once again, the glass has always spilled over for me. My let downs have always come from other people questioning my capabilities. I have a habit of remembering every negative comment that I've heard and how I can prove them wrong.

I can go on and on talking about my achievements, like my recent TEDx Talk, being published in the Los Angeles Times as an op-ed, and more than my share of fame on TV and on the stage—you can easily search my name in your browser, and something will pop up. I don't like talking about my success because to me, it's not a big deal. As I said, I never liked to be the focal point in the room. I would much rather ask how you are doing and getting to know you better, instead of reading off my resume. My family and close friends have always been far more successful than me, but it's not a rite of passage to be a GOAT (Greatest of All Time). Once the message is out, I'm on to my next project with advocacy work in the disabled community or setting up something really techie in my house. I've always been a reluctant public advocate.

When I'm sleeping, I'm constantly dreaming as soon as I close my eyes. My dreams are never flying, walking, or fantasizing, but they are always in the present and what I'm doing right now when I'm awake, like writing this chapter in this book. I had a dream about myself on the computer, typing away. I never get a full night of sleep because my mind is always going, like a hamster on the wheel.

My life passion has always been AAC and communication. Communication is the most basic fundamental right of all of us, no matter how nonverbal one is. An infant will let you know that they are hungry by crying. When we go to the doctor, we often show the doctor where it hurts. These are basic ways to communicate our needs. I see people with a speech impairment, having trouble speaking, because they haven't gotten the proper device to best suit their needs, or they don't have a device at all because they can't get funding through insurance. Or, more importantly, there is a lack of support and training after a device has been delivered to them. Because of these obstacles, there is a huge communication gap in our community.

Imagine if you were disabled and could not communicate in your natural ways. You would be frustrated, and people would get the wrong message about what you really need. The general public needs to be educated that not all people can communicate verbally. For a person with a disability, such as myself, Assistive Technology has opened more and more doors to speak.

Please don't think when someone has an AAC device that it is their only form of expressing their thoughts. I do not consider my device to be my primary voice. A lot of my friends, family, and staff can understand me when I use my voice. I like to think of my devices as tools to talk to people who may have a hard time understanding me. I know people who refuse to use any type of assistive technology or alternative augmentative communication device for their voice. They say that the device is too slow for their needs, or it is not their natural voice. All of their concerns are valid, and I agree with most of them, but, if I wasn't using any kind of assistive technology or device, I wouldn't have the same opportunities in my life, my professional career, and my ongoing commitments to boards, committees, and advocacy.

My words are coming from my big left toe, but they also need to be heard and that is through AAC. What is your way of communicating? How are you being heard?

My Community

Watch my interview with Mai Ling Chan on Cognixion's What's New? What's Next? in AAC:

Ways to Connect with Me

tim@jinonline.net

www.LetsMeetTim.com

www.TimJin.com

www.facebook.com/timjin

www.linkedin.com/in/tim-jin-004280202

Tim graduated from California State University, Long Beach, in speech communication. He has been using an augmentative and alternative communication (AAC) device ever since he was in elementary school. One of his passions is for everyone to be able to communicate through technology, whatever that happens to be. It doesn't matter what your disability is; everyone needs to communicate.

Being Original is the Best Way to Serve

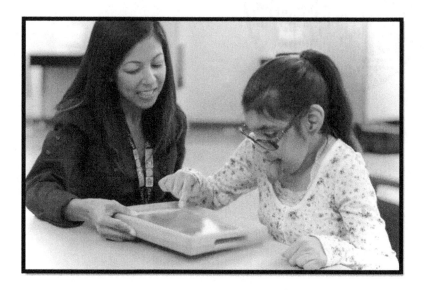

Mai Ling Chan, MS, CCC-SLP

Photo by Brandon Sampayan

* * *

This book was originally conceived in the spring of 2018. It was part of an elaborate five-year plan that involved starting a podcast and creating a series of books focused on spotlighting leaders in the disability community. I had no idea how to create a podcast at that time, let alone write a book, so it is interesting to look back now at the original plan and acknowledge that the *plan* is coming to fruition. It may seem

Mai Ling Chan

that consistently producing a fairly well-received podcast for two years and publishing the first collaborative book in the series, *Becoming an Exceptional Leader*, represents a substantial achievement and credibility in terms of commitment to the disability industry; but, it is also quite plausible that my internal voice whispers thoughts of inadequacy and paucity in the area of augmentative and alternative communication (AAC) as I add my voice to the stories of the amazing coauthors in this book.

Like many speech-language pathologists (SLPs), I received a general introduction and entry-level education related to AAC during my master's program. On my first day as a new school-based clinician, however, in a classroom with five students, who had varied cognitive abilities and different AAC systems (or none at all), I realized I didn't have the training I needed to truly support each of their communication needs.

One student had a single page with the days of the week, *yes*, *no*, and *more* symbols. Another had a hand-activated switch with one recording on it: "hello" and another had a dedicated device mounted on her wheelchair with Lamp Words For Life—a sophisticated communication symbol set that I had never seen before.

I remember feeling like a person on stage who suddenly realized she had no clothes on. The teacher, aides, and students were looking at me and waiting for me to start my session. They believed I would make *communication magic* happen, but I truly had no idea where to start. I felt embarrassed and flustered, to say the least. The kids were my saviors that day, and, for much of that school year they

197

participated in my "let's try this" activities, knowing full well that I was learning alongside them.

That is where my journey into AAC really began: by acknowledging I needed to learn more AND accepting that it wasn't about ME and my ego's desire to be seen as the expert. It was all about those kids in that room and how I could help them to say what they wanted to say to their friends.

Luckily, I lived in Arizona at the time, a state that has become a mecca of AAC experience and education. Twenty years ago, in Arizona, AAC pioneers and budding-thought leaders were just beginning to awaken their personal passions, delving into the available technology, finding innovative ways to effectively incorporate them into people's daily lives, and shaping the future with their creativity and advocacy. As an SLP who had always loved technology, I immediately began researching and reached out to local AAC experts, such as Laurel Buell, MAEd, OTR/L, and Jane Odom, MEd, (currently director of implementation resources for Prentke Romich Company), to find out more about this new world of AAC language systems. They each spent generous one-on-one time with me to answer my many questions.

Over the years, I attended many presentations and in-service trainings to expand my knowledge and understanding of AAC. I learned how to implement no-tech, low-tech, mid-tech, and high-tech options and how to decide which one is best for the person I'm supporting. I also provided clinical services within school, medical, and rehabilitation settings, and I've experienced the beautiful aha moment when a person who is new to AAC connects with the option offered and communicates the first message. There is nothing more beautiful than seeing the smile on their face, hearing an audible sound of happiness, or other gestures that let you know when a person feels *heard*. I've witnessed this with children in home settings as well as with adults in medical settings. Actually, the next best thing might be experiencing their parent or spouse cry out in elation "yay!" or "yes!" when they are able to finally know what their loved one is thinking. This is the essence of human communication—connecting with another person.

Unfortunately, I have also grieved the loss of potential when the person I'm supporting does not have the appropriate environment or team to support continued long-term growth and success with their AAC system—a sad reality. This might be due to language barriers, genuine disinterest, socioeconomic challenges, or other extenuating circumstances. Seeing the possibilities and not being able to affect the outcomes are the most difficult times for me.

During the years, I have watched AAC colleagues all over the world provide clinical AAC services AND contribute to the significant thought leadership and advocacy that has shaped the way people who use AAC are treated, respected, and served. Because of their efforts, teachers, parents, spouses, siblings, and caregivers are now included in the *Team Approach*, and are invited to learn more about the AAC device their loved one is using to be an essential part of the person's communication success. In this inclusive environment, aided language stimulation—the act of *modeling*—has been pushed to the forefront as an essential component of the learning process. By doing so, AAC leaders empower communication partners to use AAC language to *show how* instead of constantly testing the user's knowledge and limiting further growth.

The most important component of this growth is the paradigm shift to *assume competence* and *assume potential* when approaching a person who uses AAC. Thanks to this renaissance of leadership, individualism is paramount. As Dr. Caroline Musselwhite (read Caroline's story on page 1) requested, *Words from Heaven* (temporary words, hidden words, vocabulary sets you can only use in a certain location) are no longer common, and people have access to all the words we want—even vulgar ones. Because sometimes, you just need one.

I have spent time highlighting these major accomplishments in AAC because I respect their value and incorporate them into my clinical practice in both medical and educational settings. Keeping up with the evolution of practice has been paramount to me in so many ways. However, I haven't followed my colleagues into the area of thought leadership in AAC.

I began this chapter by sharing my feelings of inadequacy when comparing myself to the other authors of this book. It is easy to see I have a wealth of clinical experience supporting people who use AAC, but I haven't developed a teaching platform or created an AAC specific technology—yet—stay tuned! I also don't have a lived experience or personal connection that drives my passion in this area of speech-language pathology. Alongside these types of inspirational stories, I felt my interest and efforts pale in comparison. I even considered not contributing a personal chapter to this book, but I eventually realized that this is where my story has meaning and value to you, the reader.

I am here to show you that there are so many ways to serve, and we must not be dissuaded by an internal voice that says you're "not good enough" or "not as smart as." It is just as important to be *unique* as it is to be an *expert*. I may not be an AAC expert who shares innovative clinical concepts and teachings, but I AM an innovation expert who shares the concepts and teachings of experts!

I have been doing my part to serve the AAC community in my own unique way.

I needed to write that as much as someone may need to read it. I am grateful for the amazing mentorship and role models in my life who have helped shape my understanding of what *leadership* encompasses. As a result, I have finally been able to merge my personal talents, genuine admiration for people, and my professional expertise together through creative offerings such as my Xceptional Leaders podcast, XceptionalED, and my role at Cognixion.

As CEO and co-founder of XceptionalED (XED), an online professional education platform, I have organized and offered the AAC After Work Conference for three consecutive years for free. Working together with highly respected AAC thought leaders and corporate sponsorship, XED has provided online courses to more than 10,000 students all over the world. This includes AAC professionals, parents, caregivers, and people who use AAC. It has been our goal to support and compound educators' abilities to share these monumental teachings and create global shifts in the disability industry. I truly believe there are so many people like me who know they need to learn more to serve their communities better, and they aren't always able to attend the in-person presentations.

By offering online access and reducing travel expenses, we increased access to AAC presentations and contributed to a more widespread understanding and adoption. I have kept a quote in my office for years, "Thank you, Mai Ling and the XceptionalED team, for these courses. I was able to learn valuable information from my couch, and now I can take that back to my students." (Susan G). She will never know how much it meant to me that she took the time to tell me that my efforts were valuable to her and to the people she serves. It gave me the strength to keep going several times when I needed it. Creating and running an online company is not easy, and, as with any creation, you need to keep your reason for doing it front and center.

Most recently, as director of growth and achievement at Cognixion since March 2020, I have had the absolute pleasure and privilege of connecting with people on a much deeper level. This is related to the pioneering brain-computer interface and augmented reality AAC technology Cognixion is creating. To say that the last year has been a whirlwind of information and education in the new space of neurotechnology is an absolute understatement. Although I have advanced understanding of the brain and how this relates to cognitive deficits, this new role has deepened my understanding of how the brain responds and processes visual stimuli.

In addition to working closely with leaders in biosignal data science, I've also been able to indulge my love of technology in this role. Working together with software developers, I've had invaluable experience with software application development and explored exciting options in the new space of augmented reality. Most importantly, I have embraced my new position as a bridge to understanding the high-technology concepts and helping people have a comfortable introduction to this new field. When connecting with AAC colleagues, people who use AAC, and anyone wanting to know more, I'm careful to share and demonstrate at a level that is best suited to their specific needs and interests. I finally realized that most people aren't experts in this very new area of technology, and it is my responsibility to make it as easy as possible for them to understand it so they can reflect on their own experiences and contribute to the continued progress in this area!

In late fall of 2020, I had the honor of participating in Human Factors Assessments. These home visits were an absolute rollercoaster ride of emotions for me. Armed with years of experience related to AAC, I thought I was well-equipped to introduce and support the process. I quickly realized that this was beyond anything I had ever experienced because this exciting new technology already came with high expectations, even though the world had never seen it before.

In addition, because the people we approached were already successful with a specific AAC technology and software, they already had specifications for what they needed to be effective communicators, and our early-stage prototype was definitely not a direct competitor in this area yet. We were at the very initial phase of assessing hardware wearability and augmented reality user interface design and development. So instead of demonstrating all the things this wonderful technology could *do*, we were instead assessing all the things we needed to address in future iterations, particularly what adjustments needed to be made to the hardware and how to design the software in this augmented reality space.

This was very different from all of my previous experiences with AAC and required a different mindset. I had to accept that my role during those visits was no longer the clinician bringing in a viable solution to increase communication efficacy in the near future. I was now becoming a researcher and collaborator together *with* the individual to help further the design and development process for this exciting new technology.

But I am a FIXER! Following those initial assessments, I have since vowed to use all my experience and skills to return to them with an acceptable option. Unfortunately, one of the participants, a passionate supporter of the headset technology, passed away soon after her initial assessment. Her absence is a reminder that time is of the essence, and everyone's participation has immense foundational importance, as we continue to explore new technologies.

In addition to these experiences, I also had the opportunity to interview some of the world's most well-known individuals in the AAC community on weekly Facebook Live interviews on the Cognixion Facebook page. This was also another first for me—producing and performing in live-streamed events. Being I'm in a bit of an *older generation*, the world of selfies is not natural to me, and I definitely suffer from self-consciousness and being my own worst critic of the final product. Also, as I shared in my chapter in the first book of this series, *Becoming an Exceptional Leader*, I sometimes experience overt word-finding difficulty resulting from an undiagnosed mild transient ischemic attack (TIA) I believe I suffered more than 18 years ago. Live streaming is not the typical venue for someone who has trouble thinking and speaking fluently. But I believe in the importance of personal connections, and during the time of COVID-19 restrictions, having the opportunity to *connect* with someone you respect, albeit virtually, has been a powerful resource to many of us, myself included. So, I put my own butterflies aside, and every Wednesday morning, I invite AAC experts, leaders, and amazing people who use AAC to join me for a personal 15-minute live interview. The show must go on! I am happy to share that these video interviews have been very well received. Viewers have told me they thoroughly enjoyed the shows and looked forward to 15 minutes with an AAC VIP. They were happy to see real people sharing real stories. In addition to sharing their personal stories of how they came to be involved in the AAC community, my guests had the opportunity to share what they saw as *new* in AAC (heavily related to the 2020 pandemic); and, more importantly, their opinion of what is on the horizon in terms of technology, language supports, and services. I am also honored to have been a part of live streaming with people who use AAC, experiencing their stories and sharing in the moment with our attendees. There were so many mic-drop instances when people inspired and surprised us, with no intention of doing so. They were just being themselves, and that was the gift: genuine communication.

As we expand into future technologies, I've had the opportunity to interview leaders in the brain-computer interface industry, prodding them to share the cutting-edge technology they are currently working on and discussing how it can impact future accessibility. I have to admit, I personally enjoyed these episodes because I was able to have direct conversations with some of the brightest lights in this community.

And this is what I love to do—shine a spotlight on people who are doing amazing work in the area of disabilities. We all have talents and blessings; where we choose to apply them is up to us. Throughout the years I have seen colleagues, parents, and people who use AAC work so hard on the content they are creating. Whether it is a presentation, resources, product, or something else, it essentially takes on a life of its own and becomes the thing they are known for. My inspiration has long been the person behind the action: I've always loved to hear people tell their stories. How did they do it? Why do they do it? How do they feel about it? These are all questions I truly am dying to know!

Through all of the offerings I have been involved in, I am so blessed to be able to connect directly with amazing people and find out the answers to these questions. I am constantly amazed by their passion and commitment to the betterment of the field; and ultimately, to the person who wants to be able to share their thoughts, opinions, and feelings. In addition, through the Facebook Live interviews, and this book in particular, it has been such an honor for me to be able to provide a public forum for people who use AAC to share their stories and their messages. I have also been highly supported by my AAC colleagues and community. They have supported me with referrals to people I should connect with and critical feedback of all my work. I truly welcome and am grateful for their honesty.

Recommendations

I humbly share my journey with you as inspiration to shine through your own uniqueness. I invite you to find your light and shine it brightly!

1. Keep intimate stories that propel you to take action close to your heart because these are your *why*.

2. Explore your own interests and talents to find ways to increase your unique effectiveness and support channels.

3. Expand your circle of influence. As Alan Brightman (founder of Apple's Worldwide Disability Solutions Group) said, "Hang out with an artist," and ask their opinions. There is so much to be learned from people who think differently than we do.

4. Stay true. *You do you.* Don't compare yourself to other amazing people. You are amazing.

Hopefully, together we can make the world more accessible and equally available to all.

Becoming an Exceptional AAC Leader

My Community

Listen to my episode on the Xceptional Leaders podcast:

Ways to Connect with Me

www.mailingchan.com

Twitter: www.twitter.com/mailingchan

LinkedIN: www.linkedin.com/in/mailingchan

Facebook: www.facebook.com/MaiLingChanSLP

Clubhouse: @mailingchanSLP

Mai Ling Chan is a speech-language pathologist, author, publisher, business consultant, and international speaker. In addition to her position as director of growth and achievement at Cognixion, a leading AAC technology team, she also co-hosts the Xceptional Leaders Podcast and is a co-founder and chief of partnerships with Verge Learning and XceptionalED.

Final Thoughts

As the completed chapters for this book each arrived, I read them and quickly realized that this book is richer and more intimate than I had anticipated. I wasn't personally prepared for the level of truth, vulnerability, and connectedness that each author offered me, as the reader. I even felt a bit intrusive when I sent back expansion questions, prodding for *more*—more details, more emotion, more words—to help me dive even deeper into these precious moments with each person. But I couldn't stop reading and wondering, *What else helped them evolve into the amazing AAC leader that they are today?*

With grace and patience, each author replied to my emails and opened doors to pivotal memories that eventually shaped their significant accomplishments. The result is a beautiful collection of individual stories that weave together a notable period of outstanding growth and achievement in the niche area of augmentative and alternative communication (AAC).

I hope as you moved through the individual stories you noticed similarities with your own story and journey with AAC and found strength, hope, or guidance. For example, who hasn't felt imposter syndrome, or wasn't sure about their career path? These are only a few of the many emotions and human situations shared in this book. What is important is the continued personal growth and progress each author made and the willingness to share it with others. In addition, as I mentioned in the Introduction of this book, every author is very humble and does not seek rewards or recognition for their efforts, only awareness.

This is the essence of a leader.

Whether you are a person who uses AAC (or another method of communication), a parent, assistive technology professional, speech-language pathologist, research professional, communication partner, or student who is just beginning to learn about this area of human interaction, you also have the opportunity to harness your innate talents, passion, and skills to be a guiding light for others.

Here are a few final recommendations to help you on your journey.

1. Learn more about us and connect directly through our additional resource links and direct contact information.

2. Be inspired by people all over the world who are dedicated to the world of disabilities through my *Xceptional Leaders* podcast interviews. Hear their voices as they share their stories, visions, successes, and challenges.

3. Read the personal stories of a few of my amazing podcast guests in the first book in this series, *Becoming an Exceptional Leader.*

4. Join the Brilliance Zone Facebook group (https://www.facebook.com/groups/brilliancezone) where disability-focused leaders learn, share, and support each other. This group will provide you with more direct interaction.

5. Talk with people. For a more personal experience, join the SLP Lounge or Exceptional Entrepreneurs club on the audio-only Clubhouse app where we have real conversations about our experiences.

Mai Ling Chan

There are so many ways for you to grow and continue along your journey to helping people communicate. Just let us know how we can help you help more people.

Made in the USA
Las Vegas, NV
31 March 2021

20585393R00135